Orthoplastic Techniques for Lower Extremity Reconstruction — Part II

Editors

EDGARDO R. RODRIGUEZ-COLLAZO
SUHAIL MASADEH

CLINICS IN PODIATRIC MEDICINE AND SURGERY

www.podiatric.theclinics.com

Consulting Editor
THOMAS J. CHANG

January 2021 • Volume 38 • Number 1

ELSEVIER

1600 John F. Kennedy Boulevard • Suite 1800 • Philadelphia, Pennsylvania, 19103-2899

http://www.theclinics.com

CLINICS IN PODIATRIC MEDICINE AND SURGERY Volume 38, Number 1
January 2021 ISSN 0891-8422, ISBN-13: 978-0-323-83572-5

Editor: Lauren Boyle
Developmental Editor: Nicole Congleton

Clinics in Podiatric Medicine and Surgery (ISSN 0891-8422) is published quarterly by Elsevier Inc., 360 Park Avenue South, New York, NY 10010-1710. Months of issue are January, April, July, and October. Business and Editorial Offices: 1600 John F. Kennedy Blvd., Ste. 1800, Philadelphia, PA 19103-2899. Customer Service Office: 3251 Riverport Lane, Maryland Heights, MO 63043. Periodicals postage paid at New York, NY and additional mailing offices. Subscription prices are $310.00 per year for US individuals, $750.00 per year for US institutions, $100.00 per year for US students and residents, $382.00 per year for Canadian individuals, $776.00 for Canadian institutions, $462.00 for international individuals, $776.00 per year for international institutions, $100.00 per year for Canadian students/residents, and $220.00 per year for foreign students/residents. To receive student/resident rate, orders must be accompanied by name of affiliated institution, date of term, and the *signature* of program/residency coordinator on institution letterhead. Orders will be billed at individual rate until proof of status is received. Foreign air speed delivery is included in all *Clinics* subscription prices. All prices are subject to change without notice. POSTMASTER: Send address changes to *Clinics in Podiatric Medicine and Surgery*, Elsevier Health Sciences Division, Subscription Customer Service, 3251 Riverport Lane, Maryland Heights, MO 63043. **Customer Service: 1-800-654-2452 (US). From outside of the US, call 314-447-8871. Fax: 314-447-8029. E-mail: JournalsCustomerService-usa@elsevier.com (for print support); JournalsOnlineSupport-usa@elsevier.com (for online support).**

Reprints. For copies of 100 or more of articles in this publication, please contact the Commercial Reprints Department, Elsevier Inc., 360 Park Avenue South, New York, NY 10010-1710. Tel.: 212-633-3874; Fax: 212-633-3820; E-mail: reprints@elsevier.com.

Clinics in Podiatric Medicine and Surgery is covered in *MEDLINE/PubMed (Index Medicus)* and *EMBASE/Excerpta Medica*.

Contributors

CONSULTING EDITOR

THOMAS J. CHANG, DPM
Clinical Professor and Past Chairman, Department of Podiatric Surgery, California College of Podiatric Medicine, Faculty, The Podiatry Institute, Redwood Orthopedic Surgery Associates, Santa Rosa, California, USA

EDITORS

EDGARDO R. RODRIGUEZ-COLLAZO, DPM
Founder and Chairman of the Chicago Lower Extremity Symposium, Amita Saint Joseph Hospital, Department of Surgery, Director of Fellowship Program and Associate Residency Program, Adults and Pediatric Ilizarov Lower Extremity Reconstruction, Reconstructive Peripheral Nerve Surgery and Microsurgery, Founder American Orthoplastic and Microsurgery Society, Chicago, Illinois, USA

SUHAIL MASADEH, DPM
Associate Professor of Surgery, Residency Director and Division Chief, Surgical Podiatry Program, University of Cincinnati, University of Cincinnati Medical Center, Chief Surgical Podiatry, Cincinnati Veteran Affairs Medical Center, Cincinnati, Ohio, USA

AUTHORS

CHRISTOPHER BIBBO, DO, DPM, FACS, FAAOS, FACFAS
Chief, Foot and Ankle Surgery, Plastic Reconstructive and Microsurgery, Orthopaedic Trauma and MSK Infection Services, Rubin Institute for Advanced Orthopaedics, International Center for Limb Lengthening, Sinai Hospital of Baltimore, Baltimore, Maryland, USA

CASIE M. BLANTON, DPM
Fellow, The Reconstruction Institute of The Bellevue Hospital, Bellevue, Ohio, USA

COLEMAN O. CLOUGHERTY, DPM
Research Director, The Reconstruction Institute of The Bellevue Hospital Fellowship, Bellevue, Ohio, USA

PETER A. CRISOLOGO, DPM, AACFAS, FACFAOM
Assistant Professor of Surgery, Division of Podiatric Surgery, University of Cincinnati Medical Center, Cincinnati, Ohio, USA

CHRISTOPHER GREEN, DPM, FACFAS, FACFOAM
Director of Limb Salvage, Southwest Integris Medical Center, Oklahoma City, Oklahoma, USA

SHAWKAT GHAZAL HAFEZ HASSN, MD
Assistant Fellow of Orthopedic Surgery, General Organization of Teaching Hospitals and Neuromuscular Institute, Gizza, Cairo, Egypt

BRYAN HALL, DPM
Assistant Professor, Department of Surgery, Division of Podiatric Surgery, Associate Program Director of Podiatric Surgery Residency, University of Cincinnati Medical Center, Cincinnati, Ohio, USA

JORDAN A. HENNING, DPM
Assistant Professor of Surgery, University of Cincinnati Medical Center, Staff Podiatrist Cincinnati Veterans Affairs Medical Center, Cincinnati, Ohio, USA

BYRON HUTCHINSON, DPM, FACFAS
Medical Director, CHI Fransican Advanced Foot and Ankle Fellowship, Franciscan Foot and Ankle Associates, Burien, Washington, USA

LANCE J. JOHNSON, DPM
Resident Physician, University of Cincinnati Medical Center, Cincinnati, Ohio, USA

HAMID A. KHAN, MD
Research fellow, SpineTech, Brain and Spine Center of Southeast Texas, Shenandoah, Texas, USA

ARSHAD A. KHAN, DPM, FACFAS, FACFAOM
Volunteer Assistant Clinical Professor, Department of Orthopedic Surgery, Indiana University School of Medicine, Clinical Director, SpineTech, Brain and Spine Centers of Southeast Texas, Beaumont, Texas, USA

MICHAEL D. LIETTE, DPM
Resident Physician, Division of Podiatric Surgery, University of Cincinnati Medical Center, Cincinnati, Ohio, USA

ERWIN LO, MD
Clinical Assistant professor, University of Texas Medical School, Mischer Neuroscience Institute, Houston, Texas, USA; Neurosurgeon and Founder, SpineTech, Brain and Spine Center of Southeast Texas, Shenandoah, Texas, USA

SUHAIL MASADEH, DPM
Associate Professor of Surgery, Residency Director and Division Chief, Surgical Podiatry Program, University of Cincinnati, University of Cincinnati Medical Center, Chief Surgical Podiatry, Cincinnati Veteran Affairs Medical Center, Cincinnati, Ohio, USA

KELSEY MILLONIG, DPM, MPH, AACFAS
Fellow, Rubin Institute of Advanced Orthopedics, International Center for Limb Lengthening, Baltimore, Maryland, USA

RYAN PEREIRA, DPM
Lower Extremity Orthoplastic and Peripheral Nerve Microsurgeon, Private Practice, Anastasia Medical Group, Saint Augustine, Florida, USA

WILLIAM C. PERRY, DPM
Adjunct Professor of Surgery, University of Cincinnati Medical Center, Attending Podiatrist, Cincinnati Veteran Affairs Medical Center, Veterans Affairs Hospital, Cincinnati, Ohio, USA

DANNY PLYLER, DPM
Resident, Cleveland Clinic Foundation/Surgical Hospital of Oklahoma, Oklahoma City, Oklahoma, USA

ASIM RAJA, DPM, FACFAS
Program Director, PMSR/RRA, Department of Orthopedics and Rehabilitation (DO&R), Womack Army Medical Center, Fort Bragg, North Carolina, USA

EDGARDO R. RODRIGUEZ-COLLAZO, DPM
Founder and Chairman of the Chicago Lower Extremity Symposium, Amita Saint Joseph Hospital, Department of Surgery, Director of Fellowship Program and Associate Residency Program, Adults and Pediatric Ilizarov Lower Extremity Reconstruction, Reconstructive Peripheral Nerve Surgery and Microsurgery, Founder American Orthoplastic and Microsurgery Society, Chicago, Illinois, USA

KAITLYN L. WARD, DPM
Fellow, Complex Deformity Correction and Microsurgical Limb Reconstruction

SUJIN YU, MD
Neurologist, SpineTech, Brain and Spine Center of Southeast Texas, Shenandoah, Texas, USA

Contents

> Bone marrow aspirate (BMA) is an emerging therapy that is gaining popularity for orthoplastic reconstruction. The stem cells collected are multipotent and regenerative in nature. In addition to stem cells, other biological components collected augment the mitogen of local cells, proliferation, and angiogenesis, and inhibit proinflammatory cytokine and bacteria to optimize an environment to heal. The most common site for harvest is the iliac crest. Techniques for harvesting BMA are simple to perform, financially modest, and associated with low morbidity. Additional research is needed to evolve and standardize the technology; however, BMA is proven to be advantageous for tissue repair.

> In the diabetic and peripheral vascular disease population there is a high risk of further amputation following a primary amputation. Amputation surgery is often approached negating the biomechanics of the lower extremity leading to complications or additional surgery. Implementing appropriate tendon balancing of stump and applying orthoplastic techniques will improve outcomes. This article introduces the basic techniques to a wider audience of foot and ankle surgeons. Specifically, this article is intended to be a descriptive guide for the use of tendon balancing and intrinsic muscle advancements in the various levels of foot amputations.

> The management of pedal ulcerations is often challenging because of a failure to correct underlying biomechanical deformities. Without correcting the biomechanical driving force creating the increased plantar pressures, it is unlikely for routine wound care to provide lasting solutions to pedal ulcerations. Patients with diabetes often experience glycosylation of their tendons, leading to contracture and pursuant deformity, creating imbalanced pressure distributions and eventual plantar ulceration. This article evaluates the efficacy of various lower extremity tendon transfers to

Non–weight bearing is mandatory after soft tissue reconstructions of the weight-bearing and the high-pressure areas in the lower extremity. The most common method of patient mobilization after surgical reconstruction of chronic foot and ankle wounds has been to place patients non–weight bearing with crutches, walkers, or a wheelchair. Often patients are older, have more complex medical comorbidities, are deconditioned, and simply cannot comply with the prescribed weight-bearing status with these methods, which leads to deconditioning, depression, or noncompliance. Noncompliance quickly leads to failure of the reconstructive effort and the serious threat of limb loss.

To date, more than 150 surgical techniques have been described for the treatment of intractable nerve pain. However, owing to their technical complexity, as well as the lack of comparative studies in the literature, there is currently no consensus on the appropriate management of this often debilitating condition. Therefore, we present our surgical algorithm, based on Seddon's classification to differentiate the degree of nerve injury, and subsequent treatment course for the management of lower extremity neurogenic pain.

 Video content accompanies this article at http://www.podiatric. theclinics.com.

Foot drop represents a complex pathologic condition, requiring a multidisciplinary approach for appropriate evaluation and treatment. Multiple etiologic factors require recognition before considering invasive/operative intervention. When considering surgical management for the treatment of foot drop, it is first and foremost imperative to establish the cause of the condition. Not all causes resulting in clinical foot drop have surgical options. Establishing a cause allows the provider to more appropriately curtail a multidisciplinary approach to working-up, and ultimately, treating the patient. The authors offer an algorithm for evaluating and treating foot drop conditions associated with lumbar spine radiculopathy and peripheral nerve lesions.

The induced membrane technique is a simple, effective, and reproducible treatment method for segmental bone defects. It is a 2-stage approach that requires eventual autologous bone graft to manage the deficit. The first stage requires debridement of all nonviable tissue while preserving a healthy soft tissue envelope. A polymethylmethacrylate is implanted between the osseous segments to maintain length. The osseous defect can be stabilized internally or externally. During the second stage, a vascularized induced membrane is formed and produces multiple growth factors. The induced membrane technique is a valuable option for limb salvage in cases of segmental bone defects.

The use of external fixators for distraction osteogenesis has revolutionized treatment options for segmental bone defects in the tibia. Following corticotomy, the latency phase allows the biologic environment to initiate healing, and optimized distraction rates produce regenerate. Regenerate consolidation can be improved with local and systemic biologic optimization. Consolidation time is often considered to be 3 to 4 times longer than distraction in adults. Soft tissue considerations are important during external fixation and distraction. Additionally, slow regenerate can be benefited by various techniques discussed in this article. Distraction osteogenesis is a beneficial tool for segmental bone defects.

Reconstruction of critical size bone defects in the lower extremity poses a significant risk to not only limb malfunction but also amputation. The reconstructive goal of free bone flaps is to provide vascularized bone that restores length and stability. This applies to the native limb and also in amputations when a vascularized length of bone is required to maintain level of amputation. Multiple anatomic regions of the lower extremity may be successfully reconstructed with the fibula free flap.

CLINICS IN PODIATRIC MEDICINE AND SURGERY

FORTHCOMING ISSUES

April 2021
Posterior and Plantar Heel Pain
Eric A. Barp, *Editor*

July 2021
Cavus Foot Deformity
John Visser, *Editor*

RECENT ISSUES

October 2020
Orthoplastic techniques for lower extremity reconstruction - Part I
Edgardo R. Rodriguez-Collazo and Suhail Masadeh, *Editors*

July 2020
Revisional Surgery
Sean T. Grambart, *Editor*

SERIES OF RELATED INTEREST

Orthopedic Clinics
Clinics in Sports Medicine
Foot and Ankle Clinics
Physical Medicine and Rehabilitation Clinics

THE CLINICS ARE AVAILABLE ONLINE!
Access your subscription at:
www.theclinics.com

Foreword

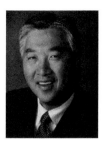

Thomas J. Chang, DPM
Consulting Editor

It is my pleasure to present the second of two issues on the topic of "Orthoplastics." This is a term capturing the essence of what we already do within our specialty, from the lower leg to the toes. No other specialty focuses equal attention to skin and wounds, to damaged soft tissues, and to correction of bone deformity.

Over the past decade, I have witnessed an explosion of information and courses in lower-extremity plastic surgery, wound care, rotational and advancement skin and muscle flaps, bone surgery, including stabilization and transport, and deformity correction. The area of limb salvage has grown exponentially in the amount of knowledge and resources available, and many more compromised limbs are corrected and preserved than ever before.

In the first issue, I introduced Dr. Edgardo Rodriguez-Collazo and his vision for Orthoplastics education to lower extremity surgeons throughout the world. There is also a co-editor listed within these two volumes who deserves recognition as well. These two issues devoted to the topic of Orthoplastic surgery are also skillfully designed by Dr. Suhail Masadeh of Cincinnati. He has beautifully edited and co-authored many of the papers within the first issue. Professor Masadeh is at the forefront of advances and education in the field of Orthoplastic surgery. A masterful surgical anatomist and dedicated educator, Dr. Masadeh has had a profound influence on both young and experienced surgeons, and is highly regarded by his peers for not only his skills, but also for his passion and drive to expand our knowledge base.

This issue of *Clinics* continues with the topic of Orthoplastics, and will focus on osseous reconstruction and updating modern techniques in peripheral neuro-microsurgery. It is again authored by experts in the combined fields of lower extremity musculoskeletal and plastic reconstructive surgery.

Clin Podiatr Med Surg 38 (2021) xi–xii
https://doi.org/10.1016/j.cpm.2020.09.009
0891-8422/21/© 2020 Published by Elsevier Inc.

podiatric.theclinics.com

I trust both issues will be worthwhile additions to your library.

Thomas J. Chang, DPM
Redwood Orthopedic Surgery Associates
208 Concourse Boulevard
Santa Rosa, CA 95403, USA

E-mail address:
thomaschang14@comcast.net

Preface

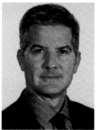
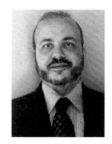

Edgardo R. Rodriguez-Collazo, DPM   Suhail Masadeh, DPM
Editors

Throughout my career, my motivation and inspiration for seeking continuing education and training were the patients that came through my door every day. I looked at each one as a family member and knew that it was my responsibility to provide the best care possible. As such, I have made it my mission to travel and learn from colleagues around the world to gain a multifaceted skill set to perform as a true lower-extremity specialist.

This passion led to the eventual creation of the Chicago Lower Extremity Surgery Foundation. By partnering with like-minded colleagues, we created top-notch continuing medical education courses in various orthopedic disciplines for lower-extremity care, from limb deformity correction to external fixation techniques, to trauma and posttraumatic reconstruction to limb salvage and joint restoration, orthoplastics, and microsurgery, as well as orthobiologics. More recently, I founded the American Microsurgical Orthoplastic Society in order to continue collaborating on more of a daily basis via WhatsApp and facilitate multicenter round table discussions and, importantly, publications. I am very proud that we have now expanded various international medical missions to Mexico, Honduras, and Egypt.

This issue is a collection of the wisdom, techniques, and pearls from some of the brightest surgeons I have come to know over the last 20 years of practice and some of my dearest friends. I would like to especially thank my coeditor, Dr Suhail Masadeh, for his integral role in making this issue a reality. As an educator, nothing is more gratifying than when your student becomes the expert, and he has exemplified this more than anyone else I have trained.

It is our hope that this publication not only serves as a reference guide but also inspires the next generation of lower-extremity specialists to continue the evolution and expand upon it for the benefit of our patients.

Clin Podiatr Med Surg 38 (2021) xiii–xiv
https://doi.org/10.1016/j.cpm.2020.09.008
0891-8422/21/© 2020 Published by Elsevier Inc.

podiatric.theclinics.com

Muchísimas gracias a todos.

Edgardo R. Rodriguez-Collazo, DPM
AMITA Saint Joseph Hospital
Attn: Podiatry Fellowship Office
2913 N Commonwealth Avenue
Suite 425
Chicago, IL 60657, USA

Suhail Masadeh, DPM
231 Albert Sabin Way, ML 0513
Cincinnati, OH 45276, USA

E-mail addresses:
egodpm@gmail.com (E.R. Rodriguez-Collazo)
smasadehdpm@gmail.com (S. Masadeh)

The Role of Bone Marrow Aspirate in Osseous and Soft Tissue Pathology

Casie M. Blanton, DPM*, Coleman O. Clougherty, DPM

KEYWORDS

- BMAc • Cell regenerative • Orthoplastic • Nonunion • Revision • Angiogenesis

KEY POINTS

- Bone marrow aspirate (BMA) is an emerging cell regenerative therapy that sources stem cells and other biologic factors to induce and differentiate cells to regenerate and repair bone, tendon, nerve, and chronic wounds.
- BMA helps stimulate angiogenesis and should be considered a strategic modality to increase perfusion of flaps.
- The most common site for harvest is the iliac crest; however, it is also acceptable to collect from any long bone and the calcaneus.
- Harvesting BMA is simple to perform, financially modest, and associated with low morbidity, making it an ideal adjunct to traditional treatment of nonunions, chronic wounds, tendon ruptures, and other pathologic states.

INTRODUCTION

Bone marrow has been transplanted to treat leukemias, lymphoproliferative disorders, and nonmalignant disorders since 1956.[1] Bone marrow aspirate (BMA) now is an emerging therapy in the orthopedic and plastic sectors of reconstruction that can be utilized to both prevent and correct complications including nonunions, wounds, and flap necrosis. To support this, one must fundamentally understand the basic science of BMA and its biologic components. BMA contains a complexity of cells including mesenchymal stem cells (MSCs), hematopoetic stem cells (HSCs), endothelial progenitor cells (EPCs), white blood cells (WBCs), red blood cells (RBCs), and platelets that together can serve a significant role in repair and reconstruction of various tissues.

Mesenchymal stem cells are the cellular components of BMA that are is most known because of their versatile regenerative properties. They are the stem cells in the body that differentiate into connective tissue. Although they only make up 0.001% to 0.01%

The Reconstruction Institute of The Bellevue Hospital, 102 Commerce Park Drive, Suite D, Bellevue, OH 44811, USA
* Corresponding author.
E-mail address: casie.blanton5@gmail.com

Clin Podiatr Med Surg 38 (2021) 1–16
https://doi.org/10.1016/j.cpm.2020.08.001
0891-8422/21/Published by Elsevier Inc.

podiatric.theclinics.com

of the cells in BMA, bone marrow is where they are most commonly sourced.[2] They are multipotent and have the capability to differentiate into osteocytes, chondrocytes, myocytes, and adipocytes for regeneration of the corresponding tissue, as well as new research supporting tendon and nerve repair.[3–5] In addition, they have trophic and bystander effects by releasing SDF-1, MCP-3a, matrix metalloproteases, HGF, IGF-1, FGF, TGFb, GM-CSF among other chemotactic factors. These factors help nourish and exert local cells for migration and proliferation; promote angiogenesis; inhibit proinflammatory cytokines, scarring, and apoptosis; and provide antibacterial properties.[6]

Similar to MSC, HSCs and EPCs present in extremely low concentration in bone marrow. It has been reported that HSCs only make-up 0.08% of mononuclear cells in bone marrow in young adults and 0.25% in the elderly.[7] The frequency of EPCs in bone marrow is approximated to be 0.007%.[7] HSCs differentiate into red cells, white cells, and platelets to form the blood system. EPCs express cell markers that bind to endothelium at sites of hypoxia and ischemia to subsequently participate in vessel repair and vascular regeneration.[8] Together these cells help promote angiogenesis, which is crucial for healing and survival of tissue.

The remainder of nucleated cells in bone marrow is comprised of WBCs, which make up over 99% of the nucleated cells.[3] WBCs' role in healing of tissue has been well established, but not widely communicated to the orthopedic community.[9] Although they can be inflammatory in certain conditions such as active infection, they also are adaptive and can promote tissue healing based on the environment they are in.[10] This is because macrophages (WBCs that have marginated into tissue) can then be subdivided into 2 phenotypes, M1 and M2. The M1 phenotype is known for being destructive with its inflammatory and microbicidal properties.[11] They are upregulated when there is oxidative stress such as with infection and cancer.[12] Oxidizing environments upregulate cytokines such as Th1 that then polarize macrophages to become M1s. However, the M2 phenotype is anti-inflammatory, defensive against tissue destruction, and actually can promote regeneration. They help immunoregulate, promote extracellular matrix deposition, and repair tissue.[9,13] M2 macrophages are activated when exposed to anti-inflammatory Th2 cytokines, glucocorticoids, interleukin (IL)-10, and transforming growth factor-beta (TGFB), among others factors.[14] This plasticity allows WBC to function based on what is beneficial to the environment, whether proinflammatory and microbicidal to tissue regenerating, anti-inflammatory, or immunoregulating.

Furthermore, platelets are widely known for their hemostatic function, but also similar to the nucleated cells mentioned previously, they have the ability to secrete tissue-healing growth factors such as TGF-B, platelet-derived growth factor (PDGF), and insulin-like growth factor-1 (IGF-1). The growth factors released serve as a mitogen for connective tissue cells to thereby promote regeneration of tissue. In addition to containing growth factors, activated platelets secrete a wide variety of cytokines/chemokines to recruit WBCs to damaged tissue to aid in tissue repair as described previously.[9]

In summary, by containing stem cells, progenitor cells, WBCs, and platelets, BMA is regenerative and inductive to enhance and repair multiple types of tissues that are advantageous in healing orthoplastic diseased states.

CONCENTRATION VERSUS UNPROCESSED

Concentration of BMA improves the recovery of the mononuclear cells and platelets, while decreasing the recovery of non-nucleated RBCs.[3] This is imperative, because

MSCs are only present at extremely low concentrations in bone marrow. To maximize their recovery, isolation of MSCs can be achieved through bedside cell concentration devices that give satisfying results.[6]

According to Schaefer and colleagues,[15] analysis with flow cytometry, when comparing concentrated with unprocessed (control) BMA, the quantity of total nucleated cells (TNCs) and platelets was statistically significant. The amount of TNCs when compared with the control increased by 10-fold (235×10^3 vs 24×10^3 uL). Platelet count significantly increased from 100×10^3 (control) to 627×10^3uL. When isolating MSCs by examination of cell markers CD45-CD10+, CD45-CD29+, CD45-CD90+, CD45-CD119, and CD45dimCD90-CD271, they increased by 3.6-fold, 1.6-fold, 14.8-fold, 4.8-fold, and 4.2-fold, respectively. When assessing overall nonhematopoietic stem cells by CFU-F assay, enrichment ranged from a four- to 41-fold increase. In addition, the quantity of growth factors that have anabolic and anti-inflammatory effects including PDGF, VEGF, TGF-B, macrophage-CSF, and IL-1b increased significantly. Interestingly, enrichment in concentration did not stand true for hematopoietic stem and progenitor cells. The hematopoietic cells decreased at a 0.86-fold in comparison to the unprocessed control. In addition to this discovery, King and colleagues[9] review discussed the impact of concentration with WBCs in BMA. When concentrated, there was over a tenfold increase compared with unprocessed and an eightfold increase compared with leukocyte-enriched PRP.

With this evidence that concentration improves the yield of biologic factors, Hernigou and colleagues[16] further investigated whether higher MSC content and biologic factors actually improve clinical efficacy. Their study examined patients with atrophic nonunions of tibias that received percutaneous BMAc injections. The mineralization of the nonunion sites were evaluated at 4 months, and the mineralization volume directly correlated to the number of progenitor cells in the original injection. This supports that enriching biologic factors in bone marrow aspirate through concentration has beneficial results to tissue regeneration.

OPTIMAL TIMING

Timing of harvest during a surgical procedure is imperative to the quantity and quality of aspirate draw-out. Based on stem cell migration during injury, it is best to aspirate bone marrow prior to starting other procedures in a surgical case.[17] Cells are at their most dormant state at the beginning of the case; therefore if deciding to harvest bone marrow later on through the procedure, one will sacrifice the quality of the aspirate because of migration of cells out of bone marrow and into the periphery.

HARVEST LOCATIONS AND QUANTITATIVE ASSESSMENT

Bone marrow MSCs reside in the trabecular component of flat and long bones. Literature supports the iliac crest as being the gold standard in people for BMA because of the ease of collection; however, excellent yield of MSCs can be found in other anatomic sites such as vertebral body, proximal tibia, and distal femur.[6] Furthermore, bone marrow aspiration from the distal tibia and calcaneus has been proven to be a reasonable alternative for MSC, especially if the other anatomic sites are not within scope of practice.[18,19] However, the potential shortcome in clinical efficacy should be considered with the distal tibia and calcaneus. In a 40-patient prospective study, it was reported that BMA from iliac crest has a higher mean concentration of osteoblastic progenitor cells than that of distal tibial metaphysis and calcaneal body ($P<.0001$). There was no significant difference when comparing the tibia and the calcaneus.[18] Although further research is needed to evaluate the concentration of MSCs in each aspirate, one may suggest that harvesting more proximally yields better regenerative efficacy, and if harvesting from the distal tibia or calcaneus, one may want to aspirate larger volumes to improve yield of MSCs.

SURGICAL TECHNIQUE FOR HARVEST

Large volumes are needed to adequately yield enough stem cells. The authors suggest aspirating 60 mL based on a consensus of literature; however, some studies say as low as 30 mL and as high as 120 mL are needed.[20,21] One may also want to consider the patient's age, as the concentration of stem cells decreases with age. Once collected and centrifuged, approximately 1 cc of BMAc will be gathered for every 10 mL of bone marrow aspirated.

Timing is imperative, so do not begin without all instruments ready, as this will impede surgical time, technique, sterility, and subsequently cause contamination to the aspirate draw. As mentioned previously, the most optimal time frame to aspirate is at the beginning of a case, as stem cells are at their most dormant state.

Although there are no standardized guidelines, standardization is needed, as it would likely decrease the contamination of bone marrow aspirate harvests. There are various techniques described; however, the techniques described for the anatomic locations that will be described are a good baseline to follow for ease of harvest, cost-effectiveness, and rare complications.

Posterior Iliac Crest

With the patient in a prone position, locate the most prominent portion of the posterior superior iliac spine (PSIS).[22] 4 cm proximal to the PSIS, make a stab incision for the entry point of a bone marrow aspiration needle (ie, 15 gauge 6-port fenestrated Jamshidi). With the tactile feel of the tip of the needle, locate the center of the iliac spine, between the inner and outer tables of the ilium. Angle the needle roughly 40° lateral from the parasagittal plane and 40° inferior from the transverse plane, pointing toward the sciatic notch. Using fluoroscopy, advance the needle with a mallet through the cortical bone and into the cancellous portion between the anterior and posterior tables. If a second cortex is penetrated, retract the needle and redirect so that the tip is within the cancellous portion of the bone. The needle should be at least 2.5 cm within the cancellous bone, but no more than 5 to 7 cm. Remove the trocar/stylet from the needle and aspirate approximately 10 to 15 mL of bone marrow. At this point, rotate the needle 90° and draw an additional 10 to 15 mL. Continue to make clockwise and counter-clockwise rotations or replace the stylet and reposition if needed until appropriate bone marrow aspirate volume is obtained.

Proximal Tibia

With the patient in a supine position under preferred general anesthesia, attention is directed to the tibial tuberosity.[23] Palpate the bony prominence and use a marking pen to mark this location. Move horizontally toward the medial condyle of the tibia, and mark this also. The center of these 2 marks is the medial surface of the tibia approximately 1.5 cm medial to the anterior tibial crest. One centimeter below this center indicates the area of entrance (**Fig. 1**). This precise anatomic location is key, as the location of the draw is safe and indicates the quality and quantity of the draw.

Make a stab incision with blunt dissection to the periosteum. Incision is preferred over other methods of dermal entrance to avoid postoperative necrosis and wound healing dilemmas. At the level of the stab incision, insert a 15 gauge 6-port fenestrated Jamshidi needle with the angle of the needle precisely perpendicular to the medial

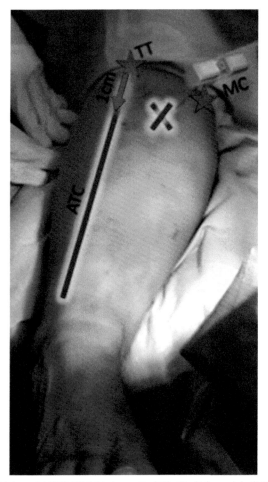

Fig. 1. Anterior tibial crest (ATC), Tibial tuberosity (TT), Medial condyle (MC); 1 cm below the center of TT and MC. X indicates the desired point of entrance for the Jamshidi bone biopsy needle.

surface of the tibia with the tip of the needle pointed slightly antero-lateral toward the tip of the fibular head (**Fig. 2**). For insertion into the trabecular portion of the bone, stabilize the Jamshidi in 1 hand and use a mallet in the other to penetrate the cortex with good tactile feedback.

The tip of the needle will need to penetrate the bone at least 2.5 cm, but no more than 5 cm. At this point onward, all of the fenestration will be within the cortices of the bones. Remove the trocar/stylet, connect a syringe, and aspirate approximately 10 to 15 mL of bone marrow. Rotate the needle 90° and draw an additional 10 to 15 mL of bone marrow. Needle rotation repositions the fenestrations to access new regions of bone marrow. If the draw slows or comes to cessation, replace the stylet and reposition the needle by either

Slowly advancing the aspiration needle another 1 to 2 cm (cm) along the same trajectory with small clockwise and counterclockwise rotations

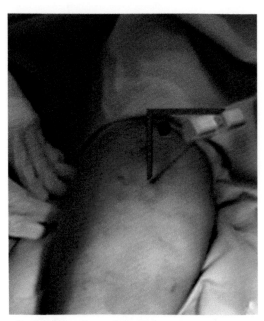

Fig. 2. Angle 90° to the medial surface of the tibia.

Withdrawal of the needle enough, staying within the marrow cavity, to reinsert downward at a new trajectory at approximately 25° anterior or posterior

Repeat until the desired total BMA volume is obtained. If there are air bubbles, decrease the rate at which the aspiration is drawn and control the amount of back pressure preferred.

Calcaneus

With attention directed to the lateral aspect of the calcaneus, place the thumb on the insertion of the Achilles tendon and index finger of the same hand on the origin of the plantar fascia to create a semicircle with the arch of the hand.[23,24] Complete the semicircle with a marker along the lateral aspect of the calcaneus. The center point of this semicircular line is the location for the insertion of the BMA needle (**Fig. 3**). Make a stab incision at this location and then insert the BMA needle perpendicular to the lateral calcaneal wall with either twisting motion or a mallet. The needle should penetrate the cortex approximately 0.5 cm. Remove the trocar/stylet, and aspirate the bone marrow into a syringe. As the rate aspiration significantly decreases or halts, advance the needle up to 2.0 cm deeper. One can also redirect the needle 25° in either direction from the original aspiration. When the needle is repositioned or advanced, remove the syringe and replace the stylet/trocar to prevent bone from jamming the needle. Once adequate BMA volume is obtained, reinsert the stylet and remove both the needle and stylet.

INDICATIONS AND APPLICATION

Indication for BMAc is multi-faceted, because the regenerative nature of BMA is so versatile. Continued research and standardization are needed; however, application of BMAc for lower extremity orthoplastic reconstruction includes but not limited to

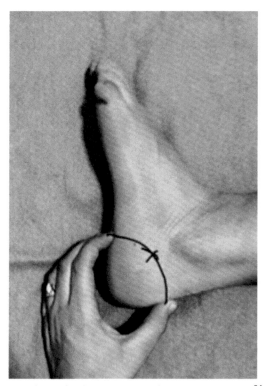

Fig. 3. Center of semicircle marks the entry point for Jamshidi needle.[24]

- Osseous repair, including osteochondral lesions, osteoarthritis, fracture healing, nonunion/revision, primary joint arthrodesis, distraction osteogenesis bone deficits (ie, unicameral bone cysts), and osteonecrosis/avascular necrosis
- Tendon/ligament injury
- Peripheral nerve injury
- Wound management, including flaps

Osseous

In 2016, Chahla and colleagues formalized a systematic review of outcomes for chondral lesions and osteoarthritis of knees to determine the clinical efficacy of BMAc. Eight studies evaluating the treatment of focal chondral defects with most lesions being over 3 cm^2 were included. BMAc was used in combination with or without microfracture with good-to-excellent outcomes in both patient symptomology and radiologic findings. Reconstruction of the original cartilage level with hyaline to fibrous-like cartilage and resolution of bone marrow edema were seen in 76% to 100% of the patients. For osteoarthritis in 3 studies, BMA was used in combination with or without PRP, arthroscopic debridement, microfracture, and hyperosmotic dextrose with good-to-excellent outcomes. However, it should be noted that improvements in pain, functionality, and quality of life were found with early and moderate osteoarthritis but not necessarily advanced osteoarthritis. A shortcoming to this study is that the number of injections, use of adjunctive biologics, and ancillary debridements were heterogeneous and do not allow for fair comparison.[20]

In regard to nonunions, Hernigou and colleagues compared 86 diabetic patients with ankle nonunions treated with BMAc versus 86 diabetic patients with nonunions treated with standard iliac crest bone autograft. In addition to healing rate, complication and morbidity of graft harvesting were compared. The subjects who were treated with BMAc proved to have better union success at 82% with only minor complications and at a much lower healing rate. Only 62% of the patients treated with iliac crest graft went onto union, with major complications including amputation, osteonecrosis of fracture interface, and infection.[22] In addition, Le Nail and colleagues evaluated 43 cases of open tibial fractures that developed nonunion or delayed union after primary fixation that were subsequently treated with percutaneous BMAc injection alone. At 17 weeks follow-up, 23 (53%) of the nonunions consolidated with resolution of patient's symptomology.[25] Considering the success of unions, relatively low complication rate, and simplicity of the percutaneous procedure, BMAc is a great alternative to other invasive techniques for nonunions.

Not only is BMAc indicated for nonunions, it should be strongly considered for primary arthrodesis and fractures, especially when the host is metabolically compromised.[26–30] In support, Breitbart and colleagues compared bone regeneration of 5 mm femoral defects for diabetic rats treated with DBM and then diabetic rats with DBM + MSC. When histologically analyzed, the defects for the diabetic rats with DBM + MSC significantly had more mature bone at 4 and 8 weeks ($P<.001$ and $P=.004$) as well as bone formation radiographically at 4 weeks ($P<.001$).[27] Rodriguez reported a case series that involved 42 complex lower limb arthrodesis for patients with diabetes mellitus, obesity, and abnormal bone metabolic panel.[28] BMAc was added to DBM powder to be used as graft to augment the fusion site. Thirty-five of the 42 patients (83%) obtained solid arthrodesis, with 26 month follow-up suggesting improved fusion rate and decreased complications when dealing with comorbidities. Furthermore, a study evaluating 20 patients with distal tibial and fibular fractures and comorbidities (diabetes, obesity, smoking, and renal disease) were split into 2 groups; 10 patients were treated with BMAc, PRP, DBM, and an Ilizarov fixator, and 10 patients were just treated with only DBM and an Ilizarov fixator (control).[26] Radiographs showed a significant difference in the rate of complete healing in the BMAc group at 18 plus or minus 1.6 weeks after surgery compared with 24 plus or minus 1.3 weeks for the control group.

Concerning distraction osteogenesis of the tibia, poor bone regeneration is one of the most devastating complications. Several methods have been described to help enhance bone formation such as axial compression, the accordion maneuver, low-intensity pulsed ultrasound, and also application of biologic stimulations. In 2014, 20 patients undergoing bilateral tibial lengthening over an intramuscular nail were enrolled in a randomized trial with 10 receiving BMAc combined with PRP injection at the end of the index surgery and 10 without adjunction for control. Adhering to similar distraction rates (approximately 0.75 mm/d), mean cortical healing index was faster with the BMA/PRP group at 1.14/0.81/0.96/0.88 mo/cm (anterior/posterior/medial/lateral) versus 1.47/1.26/1.42/1.22 mo/cm for the control.[31]

The treatment for simple bone cysts remains controversial, and lack of comparative studies remains; however, therapeutic options include steroid injections, BMAc, open curettage and bone grafting, cyst decompression, use of calcium phosphate and calcium sulfate, and cannulated screws/pins. The use of BMAc for treatment of simple or unicameral bone cysts was described by Di Bella and colleagues in 2010.[32] Di Bella compared the healing rates of multiple steroid injections versus a single DBM and BMAc in unicameral bone cysts with a minimum of 12-month follow-up in 184 patients. The healing rate was only 21% in the steroid group compared with 58% in the

BMAc group. Although only 2 methods were compared, BMAc is suggested again as a good minimally invasive alternative for treatment of bone defects.

There are several studies that have evaluated core decompression with bone marrow augmentation for osteonecrosis of the femoral head that can be used in reference for other lower extremity anatomic sites.[33] The first to describe this was Hernigou and Beaujean in 2002 who concluded in a 189-patient study that outcomes correlate with the stage of AVN. At an average 26-month follow-up, only 2% of the hips had to go onto a total hip replacement (THR) in stage I, 8% in stage II, 41% in stage III, and 63% in stage IV.[34] Similarly, in 2012 Zhao and colleagues compared 51 hips with isolated core decompression and 53 hips with additional bone marrow augmentation with results supporting the bone marrow group, which required significantly less additional procedures (ie, THR) or fibular vascularized graft.[35] In addition, Gangji and Hauzeur reported bone marrow implantation delayed progression of AVN for stages I to III at 60-month follow-up, and a significant decrease in pain was appreciated.[36] Supplementing the results, Tabatabaee and colleagues[37] agreed with their 28-patient and 24-month follow-up study that pain scores improve significantly when core decompression was augmented with BMA for patients with early stage osteonecrosis.

Tendon/Ligament Injury

Although there is a scarcity of studies regarding clinical efficacy of BMAc for tendon/ligamentous pathology, there is clinical evidence that is promising. In 2014, McKenna and Riordan reported remarkably less pain and resumption of daily activities for a patient with severe degenerative Achilles tendinopathy after 5 cc BMAc was intralesionally injected.[38] In addition to subjective improvement from the patient, at 10 week follow-up the MRI revealed improved homogenecity of the tendon. Furthermore, Hernigou and colleagues[39] evaluated short- and long-term effectiveness of rotator cuff tears for 45 patients with and without BMAc supplementation. Of the patients with BMAc supplementation, 45 of 45 patients healed versus 30 of 45 without BMAc at 6 months follow-up. Assessing long-term efficacy based on recurrence within 10 years follow-up, 39 of 45 of the repaired rotator cuff tears in the BMAc-treated group remained intact versus 20 of 45 of the repaired tears without BMAc. This suggests tendon integrity up to 10 years can be improved by a single BMAc injection.[39]

Peripheral Nerve Injury

Within the past few years, many advances have developed to optimize repair of peripheral nerve injuries without sacrificing other healthy functioning nerves including synthetic nerve conduits permeated with Schwann and stem cells. Repair depends on the transformation of Schwann cell phenotypes, activation of macrophages, and neurovascular regeneration.[40] Although these new advances are improving clinical outcomes for peripheral nerve injuries, outcomes can still be improved. Novel to therapeutic strategies for peripheral nerve injuries is bone marrow aspirated MSC-derived exosomes as described by Dong and colleagues[40] in 2019. It has been discovered that the exosomes secreted from MSCs shuttle bioactive components (eg, proteins, lipids, mRNA, miRNA, lncRNA, circRNA, and DNA) that mediate axonal outgrowth, modulate neuroinflammation, and facilitate neurovascularization. With this novel finding, it is encouraging that MSC exosomes can be used to treat peripheral nerve injury and thereby support BMA as a therapeutic strategy to promote peripheral nerve regeneration. Although further research is necessitated, the authors have been injecting BMAc within and around the epineurium of peripheral nerves following neurolysis and anastomosis with promising outcomes.

Wound Management

The development of stem cell therapy for wound healing is gaining attention. MSCs' ability to differentiate into skin cells and promote angiogenesis is accelerating wound healing and gaining great favor for both acute and chronic skin injuries such as resistant diabetic skin ulcers and burns. The reason for this is that bone marrow-derived MSCs synthesize higher amounts of collagen, growth factors, and angiogenic factors compared with native dermal fibroblasts.[41] Several studies have been conducted in evidence of the expedition of wound healing with BMA. Ichioka and colleagues[42] in 2005 studied the microcirculation of mice after bone marrow-impregnated collagen was applied to wounds. Compared with a control saline-impregnated collagen matrix group, the rate in functional capillary density during wound healing was significantly increased in the bone marrow group on days 3, 5, and 7. In addition, Badiavas and Falanga published satisfactory results for 3 patients with chronic wounds that failed conventional treatment for over 1 year after direct application of bone marrow-derived cells. They noted a decrease in wound size and increase in vascularity for all 3 of their patients.[43] Another study evaluating treatment of chronic diabetic foot ulcers with a single application of bone marrow-impregnated collagen matrix plus injection of BMA around the wound edge showed a significant decrease in wound size and an increase in dermal thickness for all patients at days 1, 7, and 17.[44]

Specifically with flaps for wound reconstruction, many modalities have been explored in attempt to maximize angiogenesis of flaps, with surgical delay being the most effective method to date. Surgical delay involves incising the flap edges and undermining the tissue to create partial elevation 7 to 14 days before elevating and inset of the flap.[45–49] This technique has been shown to introduce transient ischemia to the area, causing increased blood flow through vasodilation of existing vessels, and angiogenesis to the dermal and subdermal plexus, increasing viability of the flap.

To build on the potential of stimulated angiogenesis as a strategic improvement in flap viability outcomes, preclinical studies have been performed using MSC to increase angiogenesis in flaps. One study by Atef and colleagues[50] used adipose-derived stem cells (ASC), which were injected into 4 murine model groups: at the time of flap elevation, 2 days preoperatively, 7 days preoperatively, and a control group that received a buffered saline solution at the time of elevation. It was found that the groups that received ASCs at the time of flap elevation and at 2 days preoperatively had significantly increased flap viability (70.5 ± 1.5% and 60.7 ± 3.8%, respectively) when compared with the control and the 7 days preoperatively groups (31.5 ± 3% and 33.7 ± 3% respectively).[50] The author attributes this to the first 2 groups having a nearly fourfold measurable increase in vascular endothelial growth factor (VEGF).

In addition, Rodriguez Collazo and colleagues[51] retrospectively analyzed a combination approach with regenerative medicine in plastic limb reconstruction for 17 patients with full-thickness wounds that were treated greater than 11 months and recommended amputation before referral. All cases were treated with a muscle flap, BMAc, PRP, INTEGRA wound matrix, vacuum-assisted closure, and split-thickness skin graft. All patients healed, and it can be suggested that clinical efficacy of several wound strategies for their synergistic combination is superior to stand-alone therapies. In regards to the BMAc, the authors believe the stem cells and growth factors were useful in the prevention of muscle necrosis and for providing a more suitable host microenvironment for the skin substitute by enhancing vascularization, collagen synthesis, and cellular infiltration.[51] The additional stem cells and growth factors potentially improved the ability of the negative-pressure wound therapy to increase angiogenesis and initiate the healing cascade. Previously, the authors applied a skin graft on the same day of the surgery; however, they have changed their protocol to delay the skin graft utilizing the autologous therapies to prepare the wound site for better take of the graft. In summary, the interest in BMA as an adjunct to flap elevation stems from bone marrow-derived cells having paracrine factors, ability to stabilize vessels, and immunomodulate chronic inflammatory states.[52,53] Also, the beneficial effects of utilizing bone marrow extends beyond what can be attributed to MSCs with an expanding list of stimulatory cells and angiogenic growth factors that has been characterized in the past several years.[54–56]

COMPLICATIONS/CONTRAINDICATIONS

According to multiple literature sources, the complication rate is low; however, adverse events to consider include hemorrhage, nerve-related injury, infection, wound-healing complications, chronic pain, and iatrogenic fracture.[3,18,57–61]

In 2001, Bain conducted the largest survey examining bone marrow biopsy morbidity with approximately 20,000 patients. Only 16 adverse events were recorded, with the complication rate being 0.08%. Eleven of the 16 adverse events were hemorrhage, making it the most frequent and serious adverse event.[57] The risk of hemorrhage significantly increased with diagnosis of a myeloproliferative disorder, aspirin treatment, platelet dysfunctions, thrombocytopenia, and obesity. The remainder of the adverse events recorded included infection successfully treated with antibiotics (2), chronic pain (2), and a serious leak (1). Nonetheless, these biopsies were taken by hematologists from the posterior iliac crest and not necessarily lower extremity-focused, although those should be considered.

For the lower extremity, potential complications were examined by Roukis and colleagues[58] in a cohort study in 2009. Out of 530 patients who had bone marrow aspirated from proximal medial tibial metaphysis, distal medial tibial metaphysis, medial malleolus, lateral calcaneus, and medial calcaneus, there were no complications recorded. This included absence of nerve-related injury, infection, wound-healing complications, or iatrogenic fracture.

Persistent pain at the harvest site is a concern for surgeons and patients. A survey in 40 patients was evaluated by Daigre and colleagues,[18] who utilized BMA as an adjunct therapy to primary foot and ankle surgery harvested from either the ipsilateral iliac crest, distal tibia, or calcaneus. With outcome measures based on the visual analog scale (VIS) pain score at 2, 4, 8, and 12 weeks, the calcaneus (20.8) was significantly more painful compared with the distal tibia (7.7) and iliac crest (4.2) when averaged. Fortunately all sites improved by the 12-week follow-up, including the calcaneus, with largely unappreciable pain for the patients (iliac crest, 3.1; distal tibia, 5.3; and calcaneus, 13.9).

With intraosseous administration such with bone defect treatment, another potential concern to consider is fat embolism. Although it has not been documented in any human trials, animal studies have shown fat globules in dogs' lungs postmortem.[60]

Lastly, a theoretic concern is that the stem cells could divide into oncologic cells based on Breitbach and colleagues'[61] myocardial infarction study, which showed that the developmental fate of BM-derived stem cells are not restricted by the surrounding tissue.

There are no absolute contraindications for BMAc; however, considering the complications noted previously, relative contraindications for BMAc can be argued to include patients with bleeding risk factors, weakened immune system, chronic pain patients, cardiac stunt history with intraosseous administration, and patients at risk with anesthesia. Obesity can be considered a relative contraindication because of difficulty in finding the safe zone for harvest site; however, with the use of intraoperative fluoroscopy, the risk is minimal to none.

Overall, autogenous BMA harvest is relatively safe and minimally invasive as long as the safety zones to an anatomic site are respected, and bleeding risks are considered. Although it cannot be said that BMA does not come without risks, the potential to improve healing of bone and soft tissue in the lower extremity with BMAc is advantageous and often outweighs the risks. Furthermore, if one is a podiatric foot and ankle surgeon and have scope to harvest from the tibia, this is more advantageous to minimize pain and improve the concentration of stem cells collected.

COMPARISON OF BONE MARROW ASPIRATE VERSUS PLATELET-RICH PLASMA

The large difference from BMAc and platelet-rich-plasma (PRP) is that BMAc has stem cells plus additional growth factors that are not secreted from platelets. PRP, as its name implies, provides the ability for regeneration through the excretion of growth factors from platelets and recruitment of WBCs. The growth factors released serve as a mitogen for connective tissue cells and other cells to thereby promote generation of tissue. BMAc has the additional potential to differentiate into tissue itself with the stem cell collection. BMAc is mostly advantageous over PRP; however, increased risks including harvest-associated morbidity should be considered with each patient selection, although risk level is low.

SUMMARY

BMA is an emerging therapy that is gaining popularity for orthoplastic reconstruction. The stem cells collected are multipotent and regenerative in nature, allowing osseous and soft tissues to increasingly self-renew and repair. In addition to the stem cells' differentiation ability, the other biological components such as WBCs and growth factors further augment the mitogen of local cells, proliferation, angiogenesis; they also inhibit proinflammatory cytokine and bacteria to optimize an environment for healing. The most common site for harvest is the iliac crest; however, it is also acceptable to collect from the distal femur, proximal tibia, distal tibia, and calcaneus in the lower extremity. The techniques described to harvest BMA are simple to perform, financially modest, and associated with low morbidity, making them an ideal adjunct to traditional treatment of nonunions, chronic wounds, tendon ruptures, and other pathologic states. Additional research is needed to evolve and standardize the technology based on much of current literature limited to animal studies; however, BMA is proven to be advantageous to tissue repair and should be considered, especially in high-risk patients.

CLINICAL CARE POINTS

- BMA is an emerging cell regenerative therapy that sources stem cells, progenitor cells, growth factors, WBCs, and platelets for cell induction and differentiation to help regenerate and repair bone, tendon, nerve, and chronic wounds. It helps stimulate angiogenesis and should be considered a strategic modality to increase perfusion of flaps.
- The most common site for harvest is the iliac crest; however, it is also acceptable to collect from any long bone and the calcaneus. It is best to aspirate bone marrow prior to starting the index procedure to increase quantity of stem cells collected.

- Stem cells only make up 0.001% of the cells in BMA; because of the limited amount, evidence supports that concentration has beneficial results to tissue regeneration. BMA harvest is relatively safe and minimally invasive; however, one should respect the safety zones to an anatomic site and consider bleeding risks.

DISCLOSURE

The authors have nothing to disclose.

REFERENCES

1. Niederwieser D, Baldomero H, Szer J, et al. Hematopoietic stem cell transplantation activity worldwide in 2012 and a SWOT analysis of the Worldwide Network for blood and marrow transplantation group including the global survery. Bone Marrow Transplant 2016;51(6):778–85.
2. Pittenger MF, Mackay AM, Beck SC, et al. Multilineage potential of adult human mesenchymal stem cells. Science 1999;284(5411):143–7.
3. Imam MA, Holton J, Ernstbrunner L, et al. A systemic review of the clinical applications and complications of bone marrow aspirate concentrate in management of bone defects and unions. Int Orthop 2017;41(11):2213–20.
4. Gulotta LV, Kovacevic D, Ehteshami JR, et al. Application of bone marrow-derived mesenchymal stem cells in a rotator cuff repair model. Am J Sports Med 2009;37(11):2126–33.
5. Baksh D, Solng L, Tun RS. Adult mesenchymal stem cells: characterization, differentiation, and application in cell and gene therapy. J Cell Mol Med 2004;8(3):301–16.
6. McDaniel JS, Antebi B, Pilia M, et al. Quantitative assessment of optimal bone marrow site for the isolation of porcine mesenchymal stem cells. Stem Cells Int 2017;2017:183690.
7. Pang WW, Price EA, Sahoo D. Human bone marrow hematopoietic stem cells are increased in frequency and myeloid-biased with age. Proc Natl Acad Sci U S A 2011;108(50):20012–7.
8. Yoder M. Human endothelial progenitor cells. Cold Spring Harb Perspect Med 2012;2(7):1–14.
9. King W, Toler K, Woodell-May J. Role of white blood cells in blood- and bone marrow-based autologous therapies. Biomed Res Int 2018;6510842:1–8.
10. King WJ, Steckbeck K, O'Shaughnessey KM, et al. Effect of preparation technique on anti-inflammatory properties of autologous therapies. Orthopaedic Research Society. Warsaw (IN): Biomet; 2015.
11. Laskin DL, Sunil VR, Gardner CR, et al. Macrophages and tissue injury: agents of defense or destruction? Annu Rev Pharmacol Toxicol 2011;51:267–88.
12. Kaplan M, Shur A, Tendler Y. M1 macrophages but not M2 macrophages are characterized by upregulation of CRP expression via activation of NFkB: a possible role for Ox-LDL in macrophage polarization. Inflammation 2018;41(4):1477–87.
13. Martinez FO, Gordon S. The M1 and M2 paradigm of macrophage activation: time for reassessment. F1000Prime Rep 2014;6(2):288–94.
14. Sanjurjo L, Aran G, Tellez E, et al. CD5L promotes M2 macrophage polarization through autophagy-mediated upregulation of ID3. Front Immunol 2019;9:480.

15. Schafer R, DeBaun MR, Fleck E, et al. Quantitation of progenitor cell populations and growth factors after bone marrow aspirate concentration. J Transl Med 2019; 17:115.
16. Hernigou P, Poignard A, Manicom O, et al. The use of percutaneous autologous bone marrow transplantation in nonunion and avascular necrosis of bone. J Bone Joint Surg Br 2005;87(7):896–902.
17. Lucas BD, Perez LM, Galvez BG. Importance and regulation of adult stem cell migration. J Cell Mol Med 2018;22(2):746–54.
18. Daigre J, DeMill SL, Hyer CF. Assessment of bone marrow aspiration site pain in foot and ankle surgery. Foot Ankle Spec 2015;9(3):215–7.
19. Li C, Kilpatric CD, Smith S, et al. Assessment of mesenchymal stem cells in bone marrow aspirate from human calcaneus. J Foot Ankle Surg 2017;56(1):42–6.
20. Chahla J, Dean C, Moatshe G, et al. Concentrated bone marrow aspirate for the treatment of chondral injuries and osteoarthritis of the knee: a systemic review of outcomes. Orthop J Sports Med 2016;4(1). 2325967115625481.
21. Gianakos AL, Sun L, Patel JN, et al. Clinical application of concentrated bone marrow aspirate in orthopaedics: a systematic review. World J Orthop 2017; 8(6):491–506.
22. Hernigou P, Guissou I, Homma Y, et al. Percuataneous injection of bone marrow mesenchymal stem cells for ankle non-unions decreases complications in patients with diabetes. Int Orthop 2015;39(8):1639–1643..
23. Miller TJ, Rodriguez-Collazo E, Frania SJ. Regenerative surgery & intra-operative protocols utilizing bone marrow aspirate concentrate in microsurgical & limb reconstruction. Int J Orthoplastic Surg 2019;2(2):39–46.
24. Schweinberger MH, Roukis TS. Percutaneous autologous bone marrow harvest from the calcaneus and proximal tibia: surgical technique. J Foot Ankle Surg 2007;46(5):411–4.
25. Le Nail LR, Stanovici J, Fournier J, et al. Percutaneous grafting with bone marrow autologous concentrate for open tibia fracture: analysis of forty three cases and literature review. Int Orthop 2014;38:1845–53.
26. Rodriguez-Collazo ER, Urso ML. Combined use of the Ilizarov method, concentrated bone marrow aspirate (cBMA), and platelet-rich plasma (PRP_ to expedite healing of bimalleolar fractures. Strategies Trauma Limb Reconstr 2015;10: 161–6.
27. Breitbart EA, Meade S, Avad V. Mesenchymal stem cells accelerates bone allograft incorporation in the presence of diabetes mellitus. J Orthop Res 2010;28(7): 942–9.
28. Rodriguez ER. Bone marrow concentrate enriched in platelet growth factors combined with de-mineralized bone matrix for complex revision and complex lower limb arthrodesis. Orthoped Rheumatol Open Access J 2015;1(2):001–2.
29. Rodriguez-Collazo ER. Combined use of the Illizarov method, concentrated bone marrow aspirate. Orthopedics Rheumatol 2015;1(3):001–4.
30. Lin SS, Yeranosian MG. The role of orthobiologics in fracture healing and arthrodesis. Foot Ankle Clin 2016;727–37.
31. Lee DH, Ryu KJ, Kim JW, et al. Bone marrow aspirate concentrate and platelet-rich plasma enhanced bone healing in distraction osteogenesis of the tibia. Clin Orthop Relat Res 2014;472(12):2789–97.
32. Di Bella C, Dozza B, Frisoni T, et al. Injection of demineralized bone matrix with bone marrow concentrate improves healing in unicameral bone cyst. Clin Orthop Relat Res 2010;268(11):3047–55.

33. Arbeloa-Gutierrez L, Dean CS, Chahla J, et al. Core decompression augmented with autologous bone marrow aspiration concentrate for early avascular necrosis of the femoral head. Arthrosc Tech 2016;5(3):615–20.

34. Hernigou P, Beaujean F. Treatment of osteonecrosis with autologous bone marrow grafting. Clin Orthop Relat Res 2002;405:14–23.

35. Zhao D, Cui D, Wang B. Treatment of early stage osteonecrosis of the femoral head with autologous implantation of bone marrow-derived and cultured mesenchymal stem cells. Bone 2012;50:325–30.

36. Gangji V, Hauzeur JP. Treatment of osteonecrosis of the femoral head with implantation of autologous bone-marrow cells. Surgical technique. J Bone Joint Surg Am 2005;87(1):106–12.

37. Tabatabaee RM, Saberi S, Parvizi J, et al. Combining concentrated autologous bone marrow stem cells injection with core decompression improves outcomes for patients with early-stage osteonecrosis of the femoral head: a comparative study. J Arthroplasty 2015;30(9 Suppl):11–5.

38. McKenna RW, Riordan NW. Minimally invasive autologous bone marrow concentrate stem cells in the treatment of the chronically injured Achilles tendon: a case report. CellR[4] 2014;2(4):1100.

39. Hernigou P, Flouzat Lachaniette CH, Delambre J, et al. Biologic augmentation of rotator cuff repair with mesenchymal stem cells during arthroscopy improves healing and prevents future tears: a case-controlled study. Int Orthop 2014;38: 1811–8.

40. Dong R, Liu Y, Yang Y, et al. MSC-derived exosomes-based therapy for peripheral nerve injury: a novel therapeutic strategy. Biomed Res Int 2019;2019:1–12.

41. Chen M, Przyborowski M, Berthiaume F. Stem cells for skin tissue engineering and wound healing. Crit Rev Biomed Eng 2009;27(4–5):399–421.

42. Ichioka S, Kouraba S, Sekiya N, et al. Bone marrow-impregnanted collagin matrix for wound healing: experimental evaluation in a microcirculatory model of angiogenesis, and clinical experience. Br J Plast Surg 2005;58(8):1124–30.

43. Badiavas EV, Falanga V. Treatment of chronic wounds with bone marrow-derived cells. Arch Dermatol 2003;139(4):510–6.

44. Vojtassak J, Danisovic L, Kubes M, et al. Autologous biograft and mesenchymal stem cells in treatment of the diabetiac foot. Neuro Endocrinol Lett 2006;27(Suppl 2):134–7.

45. Lineaweaver WC, Lei MP, Mustain W, et al. Vascular endothelium growth factor, surgical delay, and skin flap survival. Ann Surg 2004;239(6):866–75.

46. Tateishi-Yuyama E, Matsubara H, Murohara T, et al. Therapeutic angiogenesis for patients with limb ischaemia by autologous transplantation of bone-marrow cells: a pilot study and a randomised controlled trial. Lancet 2002;360(9331):427–35.

47. Murphy MP, Lawson JH, Rapp BM, et al. Autologous bone marrow mononuclear cell therapy is safe and promotes amputation-free survival in patients with critical limb ischemia. J Vasc Surg 2011;53(6):1565–15674.e1.

48. Raval AN, Schmuck EG, Tefera G, et al. Bilateral administration of autologous CD133+ cells in ambulatory patients with refractory critical limb ischemia: lessons learned from a pilot randomized, double-blind, placebo-controlled trial. Cytotherapy 2014;16(12):1720–32.

49. Wester T, Jørgensen JJ, Stranden E, et al. Treatment with autologous bone marrow mononuclear cells in patients with critical lower limb ischaemia. A pilot study. Scand J Surg 2008;97(1):56–62.

50. Atef A, Shaker AAEM, Sadek EY, et al. The optimal timing of adipose derived stem cells injection to improve skin flap survival in a rat model. Eur J Plast Surg 2018;41:387–94.

51. Rodriguez ER, Rathbone CR, Barnes BR. A retrospective look at integrating a novel regenerative medicine approach in plastic limb reconstruction. Plast Reconstr Surg Glob Open 2017;5(1):e1214.

52. Bonfield TL, Nolan Koloze MT, Lennon DP, et al. Defining human mesenchymal stem cell efficacy in vivo. J Inflamm (Lond) 2010;7:51.

53. Meirelles Lda S, Fontes AM, Covas DT, et al. Mechanisms involved in the therapeutic properties of mesenchymal stem cells. Cytokine Growth Factor Rev 2009; 20(5–6):419–27.

54. Asahara T, Murohara T, Sullivan A, et al. Isolation of putative progenitor endothelial cells for angiogenesis. Science 1997;275(5302):964–7.

55. Asahara T, Masuda H, Takahashi T, et al. Bone marrow origin of endothelial progenitor cells responsible for postnatal vasculogenesis in physiological and pathological neovascularization. Circ Res 1999;85(3):221–8.

56. Takahashi T, Kalka C, Masuda H, et al. Ischemia- and cytokine-induced mobilization of bone marrow-derived endothelial progenitor cells for neovascularization. Nat Med 1999;5(4):434–8.

57. Bain BJ. Bone marrow biopsy morbidity: review of 2003. J Clin Pathol 2005; 58(4):406.

58. Roukis TS, Hyer CF, Philbin TM, et al. Complications associated with autogenous bone marrow aspirate harvest from the lower extremity: an observational cohort study. J Foot Ankle Surg 2009;48(6):668–71.

59. Hernigou J, Picard L, Alves A, et al. Understanding bone safety zones during bone marrow aspiration from the iliac crest: the sector rule. Int Orthop 2014; 31(11):2377–84.

60. Orlowski JP, Julius CJ, Petras RE, et al. The safety of intraosseous infusions: risks of fat and bone marrow emboli to the lungs. Ann Emerg Med 1989;18(10):1062–7.

61. Breitbach M, Bostani T, Roell W. Potential risks of bone marrow cell transplantation into infarcted hearts. Blood 2007;110:1362–9.

Reconstructive Amputations of the Foot

Christopher Green, DPM[a],*, Danny Plyler, DPM[b], Suhail Masadeh, DPM[c,d],
Christopher Bibbo, DO, DPM[e]

KEYWORDS

- Lower limb reconstruction • Orthoplastics • Muscle advancement
- Tendon balancing • Intrinsic muscle • Amputation

KEY POINTS

- Tendon balancing techniques where appropriate decrease peak plantar pressures under areas prone to re-ulceration.
- Muscle advancement alongside amputations allows for obliteration of dead space and provides an extra layer of cushioning between bone and superficial soft tissue layers.
- Amputation outcomes are improved by using appropriate tendon balancing and advancement flaps.

INTRODUCTION

A large proportion of lower extremity amputations (LEAs) occur within the diabetic population, and with the increase of the global prevalence of diabetes mellitus there will likely come an increase in LEAs performed. Reported incidence rates of diabetic LEAs per 100,000 range from 78 to 455.[1] Although incidence varies in the literature, an example 10-year observational study found a 26.7%, 48.3%, and 60.7% re-amputation rate after 1, 3, and 5 years following the index amputation, respectively.[2] With such a high rate of re-amputation, constant reevaluation of our understanding and techniques is necessary. The field of orthoplastics offers strategies for optimizing the soft tissue of a post-amputation foot.

[a] Southwest Integris Medical Center, 13100 North Western Avenue, Suite 200, Oklahoma City, OK 73114, USA; [b] Cleveland Clinic Foundation/Surgical Hospital of Oklahoma, 100 Southeast 59th Street, Oklahoma City, OK 73129, USA; [c] University of Cincinnati Medical Center, Residency University of Cincinnati Medical Center, Medical Center, Cincinnati, OH, USA; [d] Division of Podiatric Surgery, Department of Surgery, University of Cincinnati Medical Center, 231 Albert Sabin Way, ML 0513, Cincinnati, OH 45267, USA; [e] Foot & Ankle Service, Plastic Reconstructive and Microsurgery, Orthopaedic Trauma, Musculoskeletal Infections, Limb Salvage, International Limb Lengthening Center at the Rubin Institute for Advanced Orthopaedics, Sinai Hospital of Baltimore, 2401 West Belvedere Avenue, Baltimore, MD 21215, USA
* Corresponding author.
E-mail address: fasoklahoma@gmail.com

Clin Podiatr Med Surg 38 (2021) 17–29
https://doi.org/10.1016/j.cpm.2020.08.002
0891-8422/21/© 2020 Elsevier Inc. All rights reserved.
podiatric.theclinics.com

The goal of this article was to introduce the foot and ankle surgeon to the basics of these ideas and techniques. Utilization of these strategies requires a thorough understanding of surgical anatomy and soft tissue perfusion. In addition, angiosome-directed incisions with proper tendon balancing of the post-amputation foot, in conjunction with intrinsic muscle advancements improves outcomes. Therefore, amputations should be approached in a similar fashion to major reconstructive procedures to maintain the maximum length and function.

MUSCLE ADVANCEMENT

Muscle flaps have been used effectively for the treatment of multiple pathologies across all parts of the body. The lower extremity is no exception, as muscle flaps can be used for treatment of common lower extremity problems including acute and chronic wounds and osteomyelitis. The highly vascular nature of muscle allows for increased delivery of nutrients and antibiotics to key target areas.[3] Microsurgical free flaps may be highly beneficial in many of these cases. However, local pedicle flaps of the distal lower extremity represent a more accessible option for the podiatric physician with a lower associated morbidity than free flaps, especially in the diabetic population.[4]

Lower extremity reconstruction with muscles such as the gastrocnemius, soleus, and peroneus brevis have been described extensively in plastic, vascular, and podiatric literature. Descriptions of local pedicle flaps in the foot are less common in the literature but are being seen with increasing frequency. Recent examples include the use of the abductor digiti minimi for lateral malleolar wounds,[5] and using the abductor hallucis for defects associated with diabetes, trauma, and following resection of skin cancer.[6,7] Specific to maintaining amputation levels in the lower extremity, muscle flaps have been used in below-knee amputations[8] but descriptions of their use in more distal amputations are less common.[9]

Although much of the discussion pertaining to the use of intrinsic foot muscles is related to flaps for defect coverage, these muscles may also be partially mobilized and relocated while being retained internally. This concept is useful in the case of amputations, as the removal of certain weightbearing aspects of the foot may alter the locations of peak pressures. In addition, a post-amputation foot represents a shortened moment arm, which leads to increased ground reactive forces necessary to generate a plantarflexion moment. In combination, these factors contribute to re-ulceration of the partially amputated foot increasing risk for further amputation. A muscle advanced over an area identified as a potential failure point may reduce the probability of that failure by providing a highly vascular cushion between bone and superficial soft tissue. In the case of re-ulceration, it will provide an extra layer of soft tissue before bone, potentially preventing bone infection requiring a proximal amputation. When used alongside appropriate tendon balancing these concepts may reduce post-amputation morbidity.

Not every lower extremity wound is an immediate candidate for a muscle flap and proper patient and procedure selection as well as preparation of the site is paramount to the success of these procedures. This may include serial debridements to prepare graft sites or to reduce bacterial load. Even after careful preoperative planning and preparation, intraoperative findings may occasionally necessitate a change in what muscles are to be advanced or even abandonment of the specific muscle advancement chosen. Intrinsic muscle atrophy is a well-documented sequela of peripheral neuropathy. Although preoperative assessment of muscle bulk with palpation or MRI can give the surgeon an idea of what is available, considerably less bulk may be encountered during surgery. The benefits of only a small amount of coverage should be weighed against the risks of increased operative time. Fortunately, in the case of the multiple muscle advancements, it should not be assumed that if the initially encountered intrinsic is significantly atrophied that all others will be as well. For example, in the authors' experience, during a partial ray amputation the patient was noted to have a significantly atrophied abductor hallucis muscle belly. However, the flexor hallucis brevis muscle belly was noted to be comparatively much bulker, and so was used to partially cover the area initially intended for the abductor. As long as basic principles of microsurgery such as the preservation of axial blood supply and careful tissue handling are adhered to, the final advanced location of these muscles is relatively pliable.

TENDON TRANSFER

Not all patients undergoing amputation are immediate candidates for tendon balancing procedures. When used properly, tendon transfers significantly improve the outcomes of the multiple levels of pedal amputations. These tendon transfers are performed in phase of the original function of the particular tendon. Absolute contraindications of these procedures include active infection in the bone or soft tissues pertaining to the planned transfer site. If indicated, an initial procedure in which debridement, irrigation, and amputation should be performed and a tendon balancing performed once the infection is cleared to reduce the risk of seeding infection proximally. The authors recommend staged procedures be used if the relevant anatomy is intact but local infection is present. Serial wound cultures and fresh specimens are obtained and monitored during each stage until formalization can occur. Often a stepwise salvage approach is used where an initial mixture of antibiotics and polymethyl methacrylate (PMMA) is placed over a defect following debridement of identified osteomyelitis, and the surgical site is closed allowing the antibiotics to act locally on any remaining bacteria. Drainage often accompanies the placement of PMMA, therefore the use of drains and routine dressing monitoring is necessary.

The cement is removed 4 weeks later and the amputation is formalized as indicated. If no evidence of infection exists, the decision may be made to proceed with tendon balancing. The following sections contain procedural details at various levels of the foot related to tendon balancing used by the author.

HALLUX AMPUTATION

The most frequent biomechanical cause of failure with the amputation of the hallux is tissue breakdown under the lesser metatarsal heads. As the flexor and extensor hallucis longus tendon insertions are necessarily sacrificed in a disarticulation amputation at the first metatarsophalangeal joint, the first ray loses stability and undergoes increased dorsiflexion during weightbearing leading to increased pressures under the lesser metatarsal heads. The increased pressure under the lesser metatarsal heads often leads to ulceration and more proximal amputation. If indicated, the surgeon should perform a distal Syme amputation or attempt to retain the proximal 6 mm of the proximal phalanx to retain some intrinsic stability of the first ray.[10] This may not always be a feasible option due to infection in the proximal phalanx or lack of adequate soft tissue coverage and a disarticulation at the first metatarsophalangeal joint must be performed (**Fig. 1**). To assist in maintaining some weightbearing properties of the first ray following complete disarticulation of the hallux, the authors use a technique to maintain the stabilizing forces of the flexor hallucis longus (FHL) and extensor hallucis longus (EHL) by tenodesing the tendons over an artificial sagittal

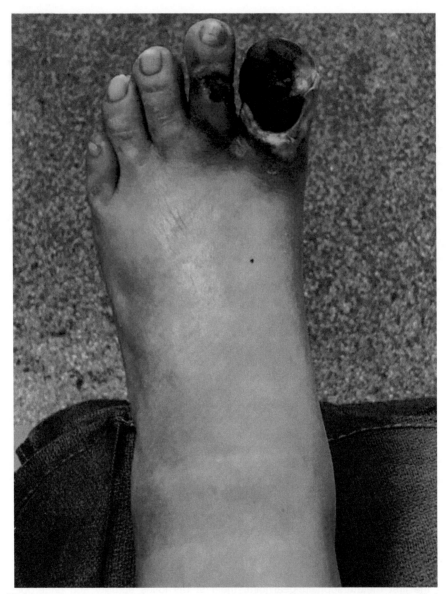

Fig. 1. Due to lack of soft tissue coverage and cortical destruction seen radiographically in the proximal phalanx, a complete hallux amputation is indicated.

groove in the first metatarsal head created with a rongeur (**Fig. 2**). Care is taken to tenodese in a neutral position and not over plantarflexing the metatarsal resulting in increased pressure under the first metatarsal head. The author recommends the following procedure may also be applied to partial first ray amputations, however the more proximal the required amputation, the less effective any transfers will be as the first ray will be bearing significantly less weight.

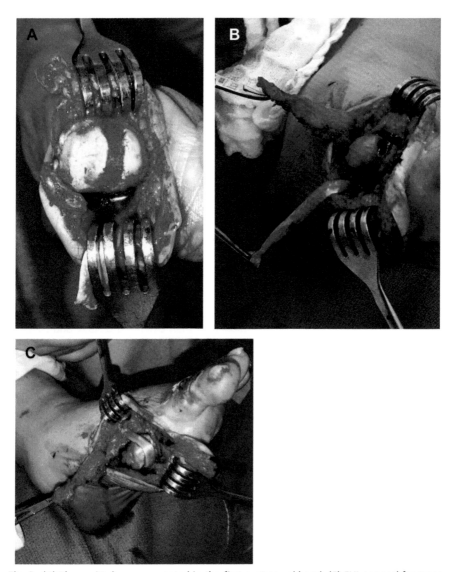

Fig. 2. (*A*) The sagittal groove created in the first metatarsal head. (*B*) FHL tagged for transfer and abductor hallucis brevis tagged for advancement. (*C*) Final tenodesed FHL.

Procedural Approach

A usual hallux amputation incision is made and full-thickness flaps are developed. The distal and proximal phalanges are then removed. The digit is disarticulated at the metatarsophalangeal joint and the FHL and EHL tendons are preserved and may be marked with suture. The site is then irrigated with 6 L of sterile saline. The site is inspected taking care to note that only healthy tissue is present throughout the entire surgical site.

The sesamoid apparatus is then dissected out and the sesamoids are removed from the site. The head of the first metatarsal is inspected and one should note intact and normal cartilage with the surrounding cortical bone demonstrating no signs of infec-tion. A rongeur is used and a groove is created in the center aspect of the metatarsal head from dorsal to plantar (see **Fig. 2**). The foot is loaded into neutral position and the FHL tendon is secured to the EHL tendon maintaining the neutral position within the groove of the metatarsal head.

The flexor hallucis brevis muscle is visualized distally the tendon is grasped and deli-cate traction is applied. Using loupe magnification, the muscle is dissected proximally and freed from its insertion and the surrounding tissues taking care not to damage the muscle. Once freed, dissection is carried out to preserve the axial blood supply of the flap including the lateral branch of the medial plantar artery, the communicating dorsal artery from the dorsal compartment, and pertinent perforator vessels as well as the nerve supply. The muscle is transected proximally to the conjoined medial and lateral heads and then reversed transposed over the lateral margin of the metatarsal head and covering that margin of the wound. The muscle is then extended distally and rotated approximately 90°.

The abductor hallucis muscle is visualized distally, the tendon is grasped, and deli-cate traction is applied. Using loupe magnification, the muscle is dissected proximally and freed from its insertion and the surrounding tissues taking care not to damage the muscle. Once freed, dissection is carried out to preserve the axial blood supply of the flap including the medial plantar artery and pertinent perforator vessels as well as the nerve supply. Once the muscle and major structures are fully developed, they are elevated, rotated, and advanced. The muscle is then extended distally and rotated approximately 40° to cover the first metatarsal head.

The site is then irrigated is copious amounts of sterile saline. Then vancomycin and tobramycin powder are placed within the wound. If necessary, any ulceration is resected and the adjacent plantar skin flap are approximated. Next the muscles are secured to the tissues making sure bleeding is noted throughout the musculature. Then, sequentially the deep tissues are reapproximated, followed by the subcutane-ous layer then skin closure. A bandage is then applied.

TRANSMETATARSAL AMPUTATION

Occasionally a forefoot varus deformity may be seen following a transmetatarsal amputation (TMA). Although the authors do not routinely perform tendon balancing in TMAs, techniques have been described. A split tibialis anterior tendon transfer or peroneus brevis to peroneus longus transfer have been used as adjunctive proced-ures.[11,12] Creating more proximal incisions or violating proximal cortices in an infected patient obviously carries risk of seeding the infection proximally. Citing these concerns as well as potential comorbidities like immunocompromise and peripheral vascular disease, Roukis[13] recently described a balancing technique for the TMA. He suggests passing the FHL through a drill hole in the first metatarsal shaft and anchoring it dorsally. In addition, the extensor digitorum longus is then attached to a suture anchor in the fourth metatarsal.[13]

Alongside any amputation at or proximal to the level of a transmetatarsal amputa-tion, a gastrocnemius recession is recommended. If inadequate correction of equinus deformity persists following the gastrocnemius recession, a percutaneous tendo-Achilles lengthening is performed taking care not to overcorrect and risk a calcaneal gait. Although plantar pressures may eventually return to preprocedure levels, the periprocedural decrease in pressure may still be of benefit. In a recent study of fore-foot amputation, 49% of patients underwent re-amputation with within 3 years and of those, 79% occurred within 6 months of the initial amputation.[14] Relief of pressure and close monitoring is critical in the months following amputation. The authors recommend the following procedure and modifications with muscle advancements.

Surgical Technique

If open due to staged procedures, the site is irrigated with 6 L of sterile saline. A scalpel is used and all skin margins and soft tissues are resected until healthy bleeding is noted. The plantar flap is advanced dorsally and if there is not enough tissue to advance, a saw is then used and in a sequential fashion, metatarsals 1 through 5 are resected re-creating a parabola to a point where healthy bleeding is noted through the distal margins of the remaining osseous stumps.

Attention is then directed to the medial aspect of the foot where the abductor hallucis muscle is visualized distally, the tendon is grasped, and delicate traction is applied. Using loupe magnification, the muscle is dissected proximally and freed from its insertion and the surrounding tissues taking care not to damage the muscle. Once freed dissection is carried out to preserve the axial blood supply of the flap including the medial plantar artery and pertinent perforator vessels as well as the nerve supply. Once the muscle and major structures are fully developed, they are elevated, rotated, and advanced approximately 90° over the first and second metatarsal stumps.

Attention is then directed to the flexor hallucis brevis muscle is visualized distally the tendon is grasped and delicate traction is applied using loupe magnification the muscle is dissected proximally and freed from its insertion and the surrounding tissues taking care not to damage the muscle. Once freed, dissection is carried out to preserve the axial blood supply of the flap including the lateral branch of the medial plantar artery, the communicating dorsal artery from the dorsal compartment, and pertinent perforator vessels as well as the nerve supply. Once the muscle and major structures are fully developed, they are elevated, rotated, and advanced reverse approximately 90 to 100° covering the second and third metatarsal stumps.

Attention is then directed to the lateral aspect of the foot where the abductor digiti muscle is visualized distally the tendon is grasped and delicate traction is applied. Using loupe magnification, the muscle is dissected proximally and freed from its insertion and the surrounding tissues taking care not to damage the muscle. Once freed, dissection is carried out to preserve the axial blood supply of the flap including the lateral plantar artery and pertinent perforator vessels as well as the nerve supply. Once the muscle and major structures are fully developed, they are elevated, rotated, and advanced approximately 90° to cover the fifth and fourth metatarsal stumps. The site is then irrigated is copious amounts of sterile saline.

The site is then irrigated with copious amounts of sterile saline. Then vancomycin and tobramycin powder are placed within the wound. If necessary, any ulceration is resected and the adjacent plantar skin flap are approximated. Next the muscles are secured to the tissues making sure bleeding is noted throughout the musculature. Then, sequentially the deep tissues are reapproximated, followed by the subcutaneous layer then skin closure. A bandage and posterior splint are applied protecting the distal sump.

LISFRANC AMPUTATION

Historically, the Lisfranc amputation has been criticized for its high failure rate.[15] The loss of the peroneus brevis insertion at the fifth metatarsal base during a Lisfranc amputation leaves the tibialis anterior without its main antagonist. Although the tibialis anterior tendon loses only roughly 10% of its insertion,[15] it's antagonist the peroneus longus insertion is almost entirely sacrificed. Without biomechanical correction, an equinovarus deformity usually results creating areas of high pressure and eventual tissue loss. The authors recommend the following surgical technique.

Surgical Technique

Nonviable tissues are resected and the site is irrigated with copious amounts of sterile saline. A saw is used and a portion of the medial cuneiform is resected in line with the intermediate and lateral cuneiforms.

Next the EHL tendon is identified then dissected and freed from the surrounding tissues and tagged with a hemostat. A 4 to 0 drill bit is then used and a pilot hole is created from the dorsal medial aspect of the lateral cuneiform angling plantar lateral. Next a tendon passer is inserted from plantar to dorsal and the EHL tendon is passed through the cuneiform (**Fig. 3**).

A drill hole is then created to the dorsal-lateral aspect of the cuboid to the plantar medial and then the peroneus longus tendon is passed through the cuboid (**Fig. 4**). The remaining stump is loaded in place into neutral position then the peroneus longus is anastomosed to the EHL on the plantar aspects of the cuboid and lateral cuneiform then secured to the periosteal tissues. Sutures are also placed on the opposing surfaces of the tendon transfers to the periosteal tissues. The site is irrigated with copious amounts sterile saline.

The abductor digiti muscle is visualized distally the tendon is grasped and delicate traction is applied. Using loupe magnification, the muscle is dissected proximally and freed from its insertion and the surrounding tissues, taking care not to damage the muscle. Once freed dissection is carried out to preserve the axial blood supply of the flap including the lateral plantar artery and pertinent perforator vessels as well as the nerve supply. Once the muscle and major structures are fully developed, they are elevated, rotated, and advanced approximately 90° to cover the cuboid and peroneus longus transfer.

The abductor hallucis muscle is visualized distally the tendon is grasped and delicate traction is applied. Using loupe magnification, the muscle is dissected proximally and freed from its insertion and the surrounding tissues taking care not to damage the

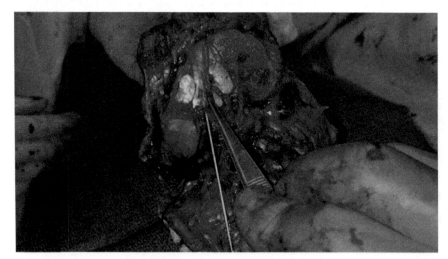

Fig. 3. EHL tendon transferred to the lateral cuneiform.

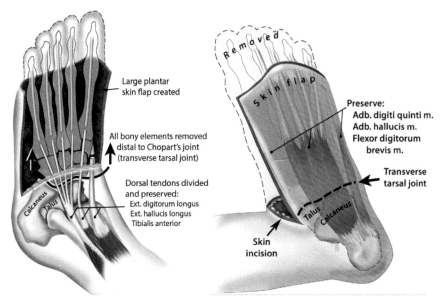

Fig. 4. A representative illustration of the planned incisions for a Chopart amputation. (Copyright 2019, Rubin Institute for Advanced Orthopedics, Sinai Hospital of Baltimore.)

muscle. Once freed dissection is carried out to preserve the axial blood supply of the flap including the medial plantar artery and pertinent perforator vessels as well as the nerve supply. Once the muscle and major structures are fully developed, they are elevated, rotated, and advanced approximately 90° to cover the medial and intermediate cuneiforms.

The flexor hallucis brevis muscle is visualized distally the tendon is grasped and delicate traction is applied. Using loupe magnification, the muscle is dissected proximally and freed from its insertion and the surrounding tissues taking care not to damage the muscle. Once freed, dissection is carried out to preserve the axial blood supply of the flap including the lateral branch of the medial plantar artery, the communicating dorsal artery from the dorsal compartment and pertinent perforator vessels as well as the nerve supply. Once the muscle and major structures are fully developed, they are elevated, rotated, and advanced back over the central aspect of the stump covering the lateral cuneiform and tendon transfers.

The site is then irrigated is copious amounts of sterile saline. Then vancomycin and tobramycin powder are placed within the wound. If necessary, any ulceration is resected and the adjacent plantar skin flap are approximated. Next the muscles are secured to the tissues making sure bleeding is noted throughout the musculature. Then, sequentially the deep tissues are reapproximated, followed by the subcutaneous layer then skin closure. A bandage and posterior splint are applied protecting the distal sump.

CHOPART AMPUTATION

The Chopart amputation has a reputation similar to that of the Lisfranc in that it has a reportedly high failure rate.[16] The loss of the dorsiflexors of the foot leaves the Achilles unopposed, causing an equinus contracture that shifts the weightbearing surface away from the plantar fat pad and toward the less protected anterior articular surfaces of the talus and calcaneus. Although consensus exists for the necessity of a gastroc-nemius or Achilles lengthening procedure, the author recommends gastrocnemius recession in every Chopart amputation along with a complete Achilles tenotomy. Although some advocate for tibio-talo-calcaneal fusion, others argue for tendon balancing through a myriad of methods. The authors recommend the following surgi-cal technique.

Surgical Technique

Incisions are planned and any necrotic nonviable looking tissue is removed (see **Fig. 4**). The plantar flap length is maintained to cover the distal and interior stump. Next the site is irrigated with 6 L of sterile saline.

The dissection is carried deep using sharp and blunt dissection, preserving all major neurovascular structures as well as exposing the tibialis anterior, EHL, and extensor digitorum longus tendons, which are tagged for later transfer. The talar neck is then developed and using a 4.0 drill bit, pilot holes are created to allow the tibialis anterior, EHL, and extensor digitorum longus tendons to be passed from dorsal to plantar. Maintaining the stump in a loaded, slightly dorsiflexed position, the tendons are passed from dorsal to plantar and then the tibialis anterior is anastomosed to the extensor tendons with 2 to 0 Vicryl suture to create a sling on the plantar neck. All excess tendon is then resected (**Fig. 5**).

Attention is then directed to the medial aspect of the plantar soft tissues where the abductor hallucis muscle, which is delicately dissected using a 15-blade preserving the medial plantar artery and perforators starting distal to proximally, this is carried all the way toward its insertion. Taking care not to grasp the muscle proper, the muscle is manipulated using the distal tendon.

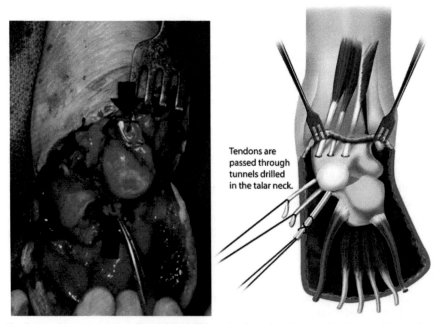

Tendons are passed through tunnels drilled in the talar neck.

Fig. 5. Tendons are passed through a drill hole in the talus. (Copyright 2019, Rubin Institute for Advanced Orthopedics, Sinai Hospital of Baltimore.)

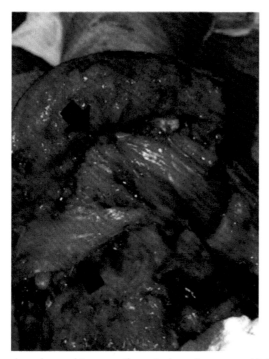

Fig. 6. Intrinsic muscles advanced to cover the anterior calcaneus and talar head.

Attention is then directed to the abductor digiti minimi muscle along the lateral aspect of the soft tissues, which is delicately dissected using a 15-blade preserving the medial plantar artery and perforators starting distal to proximally this is carried all the way toward its insertion. Taking care not to grasp the muscle proper, the muscle is manipulated using the distal tendon.

In addition, the flexor digitorum brevis tendons are found and sequentially each individual tendon and muscle are developed to allow development of the entire muscle proximally taking care to preserve all major supplying vasculature without compromising the muscle fibers. All 3 muscles are inspected and must be noted to have adequate perfusion. The site is then irrigated again copious amounts of sterile saline then the site is covered with a combination of vancomycin and tobramycin powder then the abductor hallucis is advanced to cover the medial aspect of the talar head

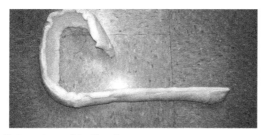

Fig. 7. Posterior splint contoured to the stump.

and neck. The flexor digitorum brevis is also advanced and rotated dorsally to cover the central aspect of the talar head and neck followed by advancement and rotation of the abductor digiti quinti muscle overlying the lateral aspect of the talar head and neck. All 3 muscles are secured to the periosteal tissue as well as the dorsal aspect of the previously transferred tendons with Monocryl suture.

Attention is then directed to the medial aspect of the foot, the abductor hallucis muscle is visualized distally and the tendon is grasped and delicate traction is applied using loupe magnification the muscle is dissected proximally and freed from its insertion and the surrounding tissues taking care not to damage the muscle. Once freed, dissection is carried out to preserve the axial blood supply of the flap including the medial plantar artery and pertinent perforator vessels as well as the nerve supply. Once the muscle and major structures are fully developed, they are elevated, rotated, and advanced approximately 90° to cover the medial talar head and tendon transfers.

Attention is then directed to the lateral aspect of the foot where the abductor digiti muscle is visualized distally the tendon is grasped and delicate traction is applied using loupe magnification the muscle is dissected proximally and freed from its insertion and the surrounding tissues taking care not to damage the muscle. Once freed, dissection is carried out to preserve the axial blood supply of the flap including the lateral plantar artery and pertinent perforator vessels as well as the nerve supply. Once the muscle and major structures are fully developed, they are elevated, rotated, and advanced approximately 90° to cover the lateral calcaneus, talar head, and tendon transfers (**Fig. 6**). A bandage is applied and the patient is placed in a posterior splint (**Fig. 7**).

The site is then irrigated is copious amounts of sterile saline. The plantar flap is then advanced then contoured to ensure proper stump coverage. Then vancomycin and tobramycin powder are placed within the wound. If necessary, any ulceration is resected and the adjacent plantar skin flap are approximated. Next the muscles are secured to the tissues covering the tendon transfers and talus making sure bleeding is noted throughout the musculature. Then, sequentially the deep tissues are reapproximated, followed by the subcutaneous layer then skin closure. A bandage and posterior splint are applied, protecting the distal sump.

SUMMARY

Advanced reconstructive techniques are available to the interested foot and ankle surgeon to provide a reduction in re-amputation rates for their patients. Tendon balancing is an accessible strategy both for those hesitant to perform certain levels of amputations due to perceived poor outcomes as well as those seeking to leave their patients with a more biomechanically sound foot following their amputation. Although orthoplastic techniques require certain level of finesse and training, they are a valuable addition to the limb salvage surgeon willing to learn.

CLINICS CARE POINTS

- Amputation outcomes are improved by using appropriate tendon balancing and advancement flaps.
- Understanding and applying certain orthoplastic techniques, such as the angiosome principle, is critical to properly performing these procedures.
- A patient-specific balance exists between proper staging of procedures and risks associated with multiple surgeries. A team approach is recommended with relevant specialists.

ACKNOWLEDGMENTS

The authors thank Joy Marlowe, MA, CMI for her artistic support with the illustrations to help visualize our surgical technique.

DISCLOSURE

The authors have nothing to disclose.

REFERENCES

1. Trautner C, Haastert B, Mauckner P, et al. Reduced incidence of lower-limb amputations in the diabetic population of a German city, 1990-2005: results of the Leverkusen Amputation Reduction Study (LARS). Diabetes Care 2007;30(10): 2633–7.
2. Izumi Y, Satterfield K, Lee S, et al. Mortality of first-time amputees in diabetics: a 10-year observation. Diabetes Res Clin Pract 2009;83(1):126–31.
3. Salgado CJ, Mardini S, Jamali AA, et al. Muscle versus nonmuscle flaps in the reconstruction of chronic osteomyelitis defects. Plast Reconstr Surg 2006; 118(6):1401–11.
4. Cho EH, Shammas RL, Carney MJ, et al. Muscle versus fasciocutaneous free flaps in lower extremity traumatic reconstruction: a multicenter outcomes analysis. Plast Reconstr Surg 2018;141(1):191–9.
5. Elfeki B, Eun S. Lateral malleolar defect coverage using abductor digiti minimi muscle flap. Ann Plast Surg 2019;83(6):e50–4.
6. Lee S, Kim MB, Lee YH, et al. Distally based abductor hallucis adipomuscular flap for forefoot plantar reconstruction. Ann Plast Surg 2015;75(3):319–22.
7. Rodriguez-Collazo ER, Pereira RJ, Craig GC. Reverse distally based abductor hallucis muscle flap for soft tissue coverage of the first metatarsophalangeal joint wounds. Int J Low Extrem Wounds 2017;16(3):208–11.
8. Brown BJ, Iorio ML, Klement M, et al. Outcomes after 294 transtibial amputations with the posterior myocutaneous flap. Int J Low Extrem Wounds 2014;13(1):33–40.
9. Ramanujam CL, Stuto AC, Zgonis T. Use of local intrinsic muscle flaps for diabetic foot and ankle reconstruction: a systematic review. J Wound Care 2018;27(Sup9):S22–8.
10. Hakim-Zargar M, Aronow MS, Gibson L, et al. Implications for the anatomy of the flexor hallucis brevis insertion. Foot Ankle Int 2010;31(1):65–8.
11. Armstrong DG, Claxton MJ. Addressing tendon balancing concerns in diabetic patients. Podiatr Today 2003;16(3):63–70.
12. Schweinberger MH, Roukis TS. Balancing of the transmetatarsal amputation with peroneus brevis to peroneus longus tendon transfer. J Foot Ankle Surg 2007; 46(6):510–4.
13. Roukis TS. Flexor hallucis longus and extensor digitorum longus tendon transfers for balancing the foot following transmetatarsal amputation. J Foot Ankle Surg 2009;48(3):398–401.
14. Kono Y, Muder RR. Identifying the incidence of and risk factors for reamputation among patients who underwent foot amputation. Ann Vasc Surg 2012;26(8): 1120–6.
15. Greene CJ, Bibbo C. The Lisfranc amputation: a more reliable level of amputation with proper intraoperative tendon balancing. Foot Ankle Surg 2017;56(4):824–6.
16. Faglia E, Clerici G, Frykberg R, et al. Outcomes of Chopart amputations in a tertiary referral diabetic foot clinic: data from consecutive series of 83 hospitalized patients. J Foot Ankle Surg 2016;55(2):230–4.

A Surgical Approach to Location-specific Neuropathic Foot Ulceration

Michael D. Liette, DPM[a], Peter A. Crisologo, DPM[a],
Lance J. Johnson, DPM[a], Jordan A. Henning, DPM[b],
Edgardo R. Rodriguez-Collazo, DPM[c], Suhail Masadeh, DPM[d,*]

KEYWORDS

- Ulceration • Neuropathy • Diabetes • Tendon • Flexible • Semirigid
- Lower limb reconstruction • Limb salvage

KEY POINTS

- Persistent hyperglycemia leads to muscle imbalance, increased tendon stiffness, and the creation of biomechanical deformity.
- Biomechanical deformity in neuropathic patients leads to localized increased plantar pressures and eventual ulceration development.
- Deformities must be flexible or semirigid to allow for offloading through tendon balancing.
- Patients with ulceration who undergo amputation are likely to undergo further amputations because of increasing deformities and biomechanical imbalance.
- Addressing deformities early, before the development of infection or worsening ulceration, may lead to better outcomes and fewer complications.

INTRODUCTION

Neuropathic foot ulcerations, often caused by diabetes, are complex, costly, and require extensive resources.[1–3] There are currently no accepted algorithms to address the cause of the deforming forces contributing to wound creation. This failure contributes to the high rates of recurrence often seen following primary resolution through

[a] University of Cincinnati Medical Center, 231 Albert Sabin Way, ML 0513, Cincinnati, OH 45276, USA; [b] University of Cincinnati Medical Center, Staff Podiatrist Cincinnati Veterans Affairs Medical Center, 580 Walnut Street, Apt 803, Cincinnati, OH 45202, USA; [c] Department of Surgery, Presence Saint Joseph Hospital, Adults & Pediatric Ilizarov Limb Deformity Correction, Peripheral Nerve Reconstructive Microsurgery, 2913 North Commonwealth Avenue, Chicago, IL 60657, USA; [d] University of Cincinnati Medical Center, Director of Podiatric Surgery Residency University of Cincinnati Medical Center, Cincinnati Veteran Affairs Medical Center, 231 Albert Sabin Way, ML 0513, Cincinnati, OH 45276, USA
* Corresponding author.
E-mail address: masadesb@uc.edu

Clin Podiatr Med Surg 38 (2021) 31–53
https://doi.org/10.1016/j.cpm.2020.09.001
0891-8422/21/Published by Elsevier Inc.
podiatric.theclinics.com

local wound care.[4–8] This failure can be mitigated through the use of tendon transfers and balancing procedures in the flexible or semirigid osseous deformity. These transfers serve not as functional procedures but as a means of alleviating a deforming force created from underlying disorder. It is well known that the nonenzymatic glycosylation process leads to alterations in tendon structure and function, ultimately creating contracture and deformity. This process is not limited to a single tendon but occurs in all of the tendons throughout the foot and ankle. There is strong evidence to support these procedures, with selection based according to specific ulcer location and the flexibility of the deformity. Although neuropathy, peripheral vascular disease, and other medical comorbidities should be identified and addressed accordingly, the focus in this article is on the surgical approach to correct the deformities contributing to ulceration. The article proposes a treatment algorithm to address flexible or semirigid deformities and evaluate the current literature regarding their site-specific outcomes.

Proposed Surgical Algorithm

Distal digital ulcerations (plantarflexed digit)

Introduction Digital deformities lead to the formation of preulcerative and ulcerative lesions, which are a common and challenging problem treated by the podiatric profession. These lesions may quickly progress to deeper ulcerations and eventual amputation given the underlying complex causes creating the deformity. They are often associated with poor outcomes with conservative treatments because of the difficulty in adequately offloading this area. Percutaneous flexor tenotomy offers a minimally invasive technique to alleviate the deforming forces and restore normal anatomic alignment of the digit.

Technique The ulcerative digit is hyperextended with the ankle in dorsiflexion to bowstring the flexor tendons. A stab incision is made percutaneously either plantar to the middle phalanx, to isolate the flexor digitorum longus (FDL) tendon, or just proximal to the web space to isolate both the FDL and the flexor digitorum brevis (FDB) tendons. The incision is typically made with an #11 blade, 18-gauge needle, or a beaver blade to transect the tendons, taking care to avoid the surrounding neurovascular bundles. The toe is then splinted in extension to prevent adhesions and promote scar formation in the corrected position. This technique is shown in **Fig. 2**.

Results Several current studies have evaluated the efficacy of percutaneous tenotomies as treatment of preulcerative or ulcerative lesions of the distal digit. The results of the studies of FDL and FDB percutaneous tenotomies for digital ulcerations are summarized in **Table 2**.[9–15]

Discussion Deformities of the toes, specifically claw toes and hammertoes, frequently develop in diabetic patients because of long-standing sensorimotor neuropathy leading to intrinsic biomechanical abnormalities.[16] Because of the failure of the lumbricals and interossei muscles, the long flexors and extensors gain advantage, which forces the toes into a hammered or clawed position and leads to a displacement of the weight-bearing plantar pulp of the toe, forcing the tip of the apical tuberosity, with a thin soft tissue envelope, to bear the entire weight of the body.[17] This area is the most common site for diabetic ulceration, attributed to the high rates of the intrinsic-minus foot type seen within the diabetic population (3%).[18,19] These lesions are often treated conservatively through various offloading measures such as padding, taping, or custom orthoses and extradepth shoes. Even with the most aggressive conservative regimen, they remain difficult to adequately offload long

Table 1
Summary of proposed treatment algorithm based on location-specific neuropathic ulceration

Anatomic Ulcer Location	Biomechanical Position	Deforming Force	Treatment	Figs. 1 and 2 Location
Distal digits	Plantarflexed digit	Flexion contracture	Flexor tenotomy PIPJ/DIPJ	1
Sub–first metatarsophalangeal joint	Forefoot valgus	Plantarflexed first ray: overpowering peroneus longus or weak tibialis anterior	Peroneus longus lengthening vs peroneus longus to peroneus brevis tenodesis	2
Sub–2/3/4 metatarsophalangeal joints	Equinus/planus	Contracted triceps surae	Gastrocnemius-soleus lengthening/ triceps surae lengthening	3
Sub–metatarsophalangeal joints	Cavus	Weak posterior compartment musculature/contracted plantar fascia	Plantar fasciotomy (selective vs complete)	3
Sub–fifth metatarsophalangeal joint	Forefoot varus	Overpowering tibialis anterior tendon	Tibialis anterior tendon transfer, STATT, tibialis anterior tendon lengthening	4
Styloid process fifth metatarsal base	Forefoot varus	Overpowering tibialis anterior tendon	Tibialis anterior tendon transfer, STATT, tibialis anterior tendon lengthening	5
Plantar central calcaneus	Calcaneal gait	Weak/overlengthened triceps surae	Flexor hallucis longus tendon transfer	6
Plantar lateral calcaneus	Hindfoot varus	Overpowering posterior tibial tendon	Tenotomy posterior tibial tendon	7
Plantar medial calcaneus	Hindfoot valgus	Overpowering peroneus brevis	Peroneus brevis tendon lengthening/ posterior tibial tendon tightening	8

See **Fig. 1** for clinical correlation.
Abbreviations: DIPJ, distal interphalangeal joint; PIPJ, proximal interphalangeal joint; STATT, split tibialis anterior tendon transfer.

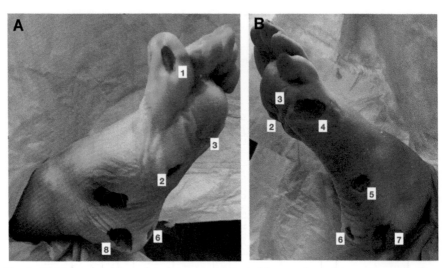

Fig. 1. Common decubitus ulcer locations recreated in a cadaver laboratory with corresponding numerical values as outlined in the last column of **Table 1**. Numbers 1 to 8 are as described in **Table 1**. (*Courtesy of* S. Masadeh, DPM, Cincinnati, OH.)

term, and tend to recur after healing is achieved. Performing a lasting procedure to reduce the deforming forces and restore the proper weight-bearing surface of the toe is key for long-term success.

There seems to be a consensus in the literature regarding the efficacy of percutaneous flexor tenotomy for digital ulcerations. Healing rates are reported between 92% and 100%, regardless of the method or tendons transected. Complications of the procedure included recurrence, shifted/transfer lesions, hyperextension deformities, and the potential for neurovascular compromise. All of these were seen with low rates of occurrence after performing this minimally invasive procedure.[9–15] Tamir and colleagues,[13,14] Kearney and colleagues,[9] and Van Netten and colleagues[15]

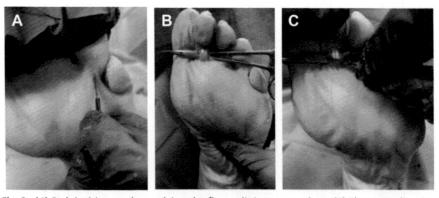

Fig. 2. (*A*) Stab incision made overlying the flexor digitorum tendons. (*B*) Flexor tendons isolated and exposed to protect neurovascular bundle. (*C*) Flexor tendon transected while maintaining protection of the adjacent neurovascular bundles. (*Courtesy of* S. Masadeh, DPM, Cincinnati, OH.)

Table 2
Summary of the literature for percutaneous tenotomy for flexible digital deformities

	Tenotomies (N)	Follow-up (mo)	Healed (N)	Recurrence (N)	Tendons	Complications	Time to Healing
Laborde et al,[10] 2007	28	28	100% (28)	10% (3)	FDL/FDB	0	2 mo
Tamir et al,[13] 2008	34	13	100% (34)	0% (0)	—	0	3 wk
Schepers et al,[12] 2010	42	11	100% (42)	2.3% (1)	FDL/FDB	0	3 wk
Kearney et al,[9] 2010	58	28	98.3% (57)	12.1% (7)	FDL	5	40 d
Rasumussen et al,[11] 2013	65	31	93% (60)	18% (5)	FDL/FDB	0	3 wk
Van Netten et al,[15] 2013	47	23	92% (43)	20% (7)	FDL	10	22 d
Tamir et al,[14] 2014	103	22	98% (101)	8% (9)	FDL	14	4 wk
Total	377	11–31	96.8%	8.49% (32)	Combined	7.96% (30)	3.94 wk

Data from Refs.[9–15]

performed tenotomies on isolated FDL tendons and showed the highest rate of recurrence and complications, compared with studies that transected both the FDL and the FDB tendons. Those studies that did not exclude toes with radiographic evidence of osteomyelitis experienced slower rates of healing, but this finding did not preclude performing a tenotomy on the ulcerative digit. Several of these toes went on to eventual amputation, but the results were mixed, with some healing achieved. Given the high rate of healing and low rates of complications/recurrence, percutaneous flexor tenotomies seem to have a valuable place in the wound care repertoire, providing good to excellent outcomes in those patients with distal toe ulcerations or preulcerative lesions.

First metatarsophalangeal joint ulcerations (forefoot valgus)

Introduction Ulcerations beneath the first metatarsal head are another common location. This area may prove devastating given the biomechanical importance of the first ray and the imbalance created after amputation. These ulcers are often treated conservatively, without an attempt at identifying the underlying cause and addressing the deforming force. The peroneus longus plantarflexes the first metatarsal and everts the foot during the stance phase of the gait cycle. As an increasing load is applied to the peroneus longus, significant eversion and plantarflexion of the first ray occurs,[20] which leads to an eversion, locking effect of the first ray, stabilizing the medial column and forcing the foot into a supinatory position.[20] A locked medial column, driven into further plantarflexion by continued action of the peroneus longus, effectively causes supination of the entire foot and the accompanying increase in plantar pressures beneath the first metatarsal head.[21,22]

Limited joint motion or plantarflexion has been proposed as the factor leading to increased plantar pressures and therefore ulceration or preulcerative lesions in the insensate foot.[23–26] Patients with a history of plantar first metatarsal head ulceration have been shown to have significantly less first ray mobility and higher plantar pressures as well as an inverse relationship between first ray dorsiflexion and peak pressure at the first metatarsal head.[23] Tenodesis of the peroneus longus has the power to remove the deforming force, in a flexible or semirigid deformity of the first metatarsal, and to prevent or heal ulceration.

Technique An incision is made posterior and superior to the lateral malleolus, approximately 4 cm in length, isolating and exposing the peroneal tendons. The peroneus longus tendon is then identified by plantarflexing the first metatarsal. A wedge of the tendon is removed, to prevent scarring or adhesion of the 2 transected ends. The proximal portion is then sutured to the peroneus brevis tendon under physiologic tension using polyethylene terephthalate suture. A splint is then applied and the patient is made non–weight-bearing for 4 to 6 weeks, as shown in **Fig. 3**.

Results There are limited studies in the literature regarding the outcomes of isolated peroneus longus to brevis tendon transfer for treatment of a plantar first metatarsal head ulceration or preulcerative lesion. Studies performed by Roukis and colleagues[27] and DiDomenico and colleagues[28] show the potential of this procedure to offload the first metatarsal head, but most current literature focuses on its use as an adjunctive procedure when other procedures fail to eliminate the deformity. The results of these studies are summarized in **Table 3**.[29,30]

Discussion The plantar aspect of the first metatarsal head is one of the most common locations for ulcer development in patients with diabetes.[31,32] This area can be disastrous, given the consequences of osteomyelitis of the first metatarsal and the

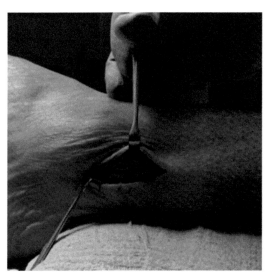

Fig. 3. The lateral malleolus is outlined and incision is planned for identification of the peroneal tendons. The peroneus longus tendon is isolated and transected. The proximal portion is then sutured to the peroneus brevis, completing the tenodesis. (*Courtesy of* S. Masadeh, DPM, Cincinnati, OH.)

biomechanical abnormalities of pursuant amputation. These drastic alterations in gait and pressure distribution after amputation contribute to early reulceration rates and additional tissue loss, which provides strong incentive to remove the deforming force early in an attempt at limb preservation.

Before performing the peroneus longus to brevis tendon transfer, a flexible or dynamic plantarflexed first metatarsal must be established clinically. It is important to establish the presence of peroneal overdrive or hyperactivity to ensure the effectiveness of this procedure in offloading the first metatarsal head. To do this, 1 thumb is placed underneath the lesser metatarsals and the other beneath the first metatarsal head or the ulcerative site. The patient then plantarflexes the ankle while the physician evaluates for further plantarflexion of the first metatarsal in relation to that of the lesser metatarsals, showing a flexible or semirigid deformity.[28] This deformity is often seen in the presence of a weak triceps surae, assisting in the overall plantarflexion of the foot through continued plantarflexion of the first ray, as well as with a weakened tibialis anterior muscle, the main antagonist to the peroneus longus.

The evidence supporting the peroneus longus to peroneus brevis tenodesis is currently limited, without any known studies that evaluate this procedure in isolation to cure or prevent ulceration of the plantar first metatarsal head. The current focus is the use of this procedure as an adjunct to others to further offload the first metatarsal head. Although neither of the 2 prior studies isolated the peroneus longus to brevis tenodesis to offload the first metatarsal head, they do show it as an effective means of reducing the deforming force and the pressures in this area. Hamilton and colleagues[30] and Dayer and Assal[29] used the procedure to further offload a continued plantarflexed first metatarsal after other procedures had failed to alleviate the deformity. Further studies evaluating the efficacy of isolated peroneal tenodesis in the treatment of plantar first metatarsal head ulcerations are needed.

Table 3
Results summary for peroneus longus to peroneus brevis tenodesis for flexible or semirigid plantarflexed first ray

	Patients (N)	Procedures	Follow-up (mo)	% Healed (N)	% Recurrence (N)	Time to Healing (wk)
Hamilton et al,[30] 2005	10	Gastrocnemius recession, peroneus longus to brevis transfer, 2–5 metatarsal head resection	14.2	100% (10)	0% (0)	Not stated
Dayer et al,[29] 2009	21	Modified Jones tenosuspension, peroneus longus to brevis transfer, gastrocnemius recession	39.6	100% (21)	0% (0)	4.4

Data from Dayer R, Assal M. Chronic diabetic ulcers under the first metatarsal head treated by staged tendon balancing: a prospective cohort study. J Bone Joint Surg Br. 2009;91(4):487-93 and Hamilton GA, Ford LA, Perez H, et al,. Salvage of the neuropathic foot by using bone resection and tendon balancing: a retrospective review of 10 patients. J Foot and Ankle Surg. 2005;44(1): 37-43.

Sub–second, third, fourth metatarsophalangeal joint ulcerations (equinus)

Introduction Forefoot ulceration, located plantar to the metatarsal heads, is another common location for ulceration. Prolonged levels of persistent hyperglycemia produce high levels of nonenzymatic glycosylation of collagen fibers within the tendons, cross-linking the fibers via the Maillard reaction.[33–35] Electron microscopy studies of the Achilles tendon have shown irregularity of collagen fibrils with high levels of disorganization.[33–36] Continued hyperglycemic states produce a stiffening/shortening of the tendon, joint hypomobility, and, in turn, increased plantar pressures.[33–36] Studies have shown an increase in skin-collagen cross-linking concentrations, with an associated 54% increase in Achilles tendon stiffness, and a 33% higher forefoot/rearfoot peak plantar pressure ratio in patients with diabetes.[36] This deformity, or change in function, leads to an increased risk for the development of plantar ulceration[37–40] and has led to an ulceration rate up to 4 times the normal value compared with patients without associated ankle equinus.[41]

Equinus contracture of the ankle joint produces an increase in forefoot pressures and is present in as many as 37% of patients with diabetes, compared with 15% in patients without diabetes.[41,42] Evaluating for posterior contracture determines the necessity of an Achilles tendon lengthening versus a gastrocnemius recession in the treatment and prevention of ulcerative lesions. An equinus contracture can be isolated solely within the gastrocnemius muscle or can be located within the entirety of the gastrocnemius-soleus complex. It is critical to evaluate for the source of the contracture to ensure that appropriate procedure selection is pursued. A Silfverskiöld examination, performed by measuring ankle dorsiflexion with the knee in a flexed position and then again with the knee in an extended position, determines operative course.[43,44] An increase in range of motion of the ankle joint with the knee flexed compared with extended is considered a positive Silfverskiöld examination and the contracture is isolated to the gastrocnemius.[43,44] This examination has shown a sensitivity of 89% and a specificity of 90% compared with goniometric evaluation and is vital in determining appropriate procedure selection.[45]

Technique The Achilles tendon is isolated and the foot is maximally dorsiflexed. Using a #15 or #11 blade, 3 vertical stab incisions are made midline over the Achilles tendon. The blade is inserted vertically and rotated medially or laterally, in an alternating fashion, releasing approximately 51% of the tendon fibers at each location. Incisions are made in 3-cm intervals from the insertion of the Achilles tendon, alternating from medial to lateral to medial to avoid sural nerve damage, as shown in **Fig. 4**.

Gastrocnemius recession can be performed through multiple established surgical techniques. After a positive Silfverskiöld examination is identified, a Vulpius, Strayer, Baumann, or endoscopic gastrocnemius release may be performed to alleviate the isolated gastrocnemius contracture. Because this choice is often surgeon dependent and patient specific, the authors defer surgical technique to the individual performing the operation because multiple options are available.

Achilles tendon lengthening results Several current studies have evaluated Achilles tendon lengthening as a treatment and for the prevention of neuropathic forefoot ulceration caused by ankle equinus of the gastrocnemius-soleus complex (a negative Silfverskiöld examination), and these are summarized in **Table 4**.[46–49]

Gastrocnemius recession results The current literature regarding isolated gastrocnemius recession as treatment of plantar ulceration caused by ankle equinus localized within the gastrocnemius tendon (a positive Silfverskiöld examination) is limited, because this procedure is often used in conjunction with other procedures. Several studies were selected for further review of this procedure's effectiveness in treating forefoot ulceration, and they are summarized in **Table 5**.[29,30,33,50–53]

Discussion The evidence for the effectiveness of an Achilles tendon lengthening has been well established in the literature. Of the studies evaluated in this review, a total of 265 lengthenings were performed and showed an approximate 97% healing rate with few complications. The major complications experienced in these studies were that of a ruptured Achilles tendon or a heel ulceration caused by the creation of a calcaneal gait after overlengthening of the tendon. The rate of recurrence varied from as low as 2% in the study performed by Colen and colleagues[46] to as high as 37% in the study performed by Mueller and colleagues.[49] Thee findings show that repeat procedures may be necessary because of continued persistent hyperglycemia and further contracture of the previously lengthened tendon. Armstrong and colleagues[54] evaluated mean peak pressures within the forefoot after percutaneous Achilles tendon lengthening and found an average reduction from 86 N preoperatively to 63 N postoperatively, further showing the power of this procedure to reduce high-pressure areas and to heal or prevent ulceration.

The current literature for isolated gastrocnemius recession to treat forefoot ulceration is limited, because most of the evidence evaluating this procedure is as an adjunct to others. The studies performed by Dayer and Assal[29] and Laborde and colleagues[52,53] were the largest and had the longest follow-up. They found high rates of healing, ranging from 90.9% to 95.8%, and rates of recurrence from 4.1% to 14%, respectively.[29,52,53] There were no complications experienced in any of the studies evaluated, likely because of the more controlled release of a gastrocnemius recession than that of an Achilles tendon lengthening. This procedure seems to have similar efficacy to the Achilles tendon lengthening in offloading forefoot ulceration, but, again, selection is driven by the results of the Silfverskiöld examination.

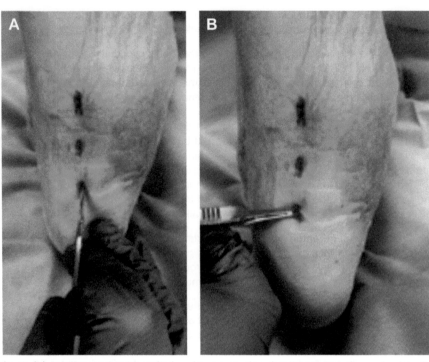

Fig. 4. (A) Achilles tendon identified and incisions placed at 3-cm intervals proximal to the insertion. (B) A 50% transection performed alternating from medial to lateral to medial to avoid damage to the sural nerve and allow adequate lengthening of the tendon. (*Courtesy of* S. Masadeh, DPM, Cincinnati, OH.)

Achilles tendon lengthening and gastrocnemius recession, when used appropriately, have shown excellent results in healing forefoot ulcerations with low rates of complications and recurrence. Because of the high rates of ankle equinus in the diabetic population, as well as the associated morbidity, mortality, and costs of ulcerations, it is imperative to correct the cause of the deforming force to cure and prevent further ulcerations. Persistent hyperglycemia often makes these procedures temporary, with evidence of recurrence seen throughout the literature varying from

Table 4
Summary of Achilles tendon lengthening for forefoot ulceration caused by equinus

	Tenotomies (N)	% Healed (N)	% Recurrence (N)	Follow-up	% Heel Ulcers (N)	% Rupture (N)
Colen et al,[46] 2013	145	100% (145)	2% (3)	2.7 y	1.4% (2)	0% (0)
Mueller et al,[49] 2003	30	100% (30)	37% (11)	2 y	13.3% (4)	0 (0)
Holstein et al,[47] 2004	75	90.6% (68)	14.7% (11)	1 y	14.7% (11)	9.3% (7)
Lin et al,[48] 1996	15	93.3% (14)	0% (0)	17 mo	0% (0)	0% (0)
Total	265	96.9% (257)	9.43% (25)	1–2.7 y	6.4% (17)	2.6% (7)

Data from Refs.[46–49]

Table 5
Summary of gastrocnemius recession for forefoot ulceration caused by equinus

	Gastrocnemius Recession (N)	Healed (%)	% Recurrence (N)	Follow-up (mo)	% Complications (N)
Dayer & Assal,[29] 2009	24	95.8	4.1% (1)	39.6	0% (0)
Greenhagen et al,[51] 2010	1	100	0% (0)	24	0% (0)
Hamilton et al,[30] 2005	12	100	0% (0)	14.2	0% (0)
Laborde et al,[52] 2008; Laborde et al,[53] 2009	29	95 and 90.9	14% (4)	39	0% (0)
Total	66	95.4	7.6% (5)	20–39.6	0% (0)

Data from Refs.[29,30,33,50–53]

1 to 3 years. Continued monitoring is necessary to evaluate for additional prophylactic release before the onset of new ulceration.

Sub–metatarsal heads (cavus)

Introduction Forefoot ulceration located at the plantar aspect of the metatarsal heads is often attributed to an equinus contracture but may be attributed to a cavus foot type and contracted plantar fascia. Although Achilles tendon lengthening or gastrocnemius recession do alleviate forefoot pressure, in a cavovarus foot type with a high calcaneal inclination angle, this may also produce an overlengthening or rupture of the Achilles tendon, leading to a calcaneal gait. Most neurologic cavus deformities are thought to happen initially because of a plantarflexed first ray, also called forefoot-driven hindfoot varus.[55] This overpowering of the tibialis anterior tendon by the peroneus longus leads to eventual tibialis posterior contracture, producing a hindfoot varus. Further development of the intrinsic minus foot type through neurologic degeneration leads to an imbalance of the long flexors and extensors, leading to a retrograde plantar force on the metatarsal heads.[56] This positioning of the foot allows the soft tissues, including the plantar fascia, to eventually contract and hold the foot in a cavovarus position with increased pressure on the forefoot while weight-bearing. In addition to the biomechanical imbalance, Ursini and colleagues[57] showed that type 2 diabetes mellitus leads to thickening and irregularity of the plantar fascia, worsening the contracture. The authors routinely perform the plantar fasciotomy in conjunction with a peroneus longus to brevis tenodesis in patients with forefoot or plantar first metatarsal ulceration with a cavovarus foot type, but it may have value in selective release of individual ulceration sub–lesser metatarsal heads in the cavus foot.

Technique Attention is directed to the medial aspect of the heel, distal to the weight-bearing surface. The toes are dorsiflexed and the plantar fascia medial band is palpated and marked. An incision, approximately 4 cm in length, is made perpendicular to the plantar fascia extending to the glabrous junction of the foot. Blunt dissection is continued down to visualize the medial plantar fascia band. Further dissection is performed to isolate the plantar fascia on its dorsal and plantar aspects, and the fascia is released from medial to lateral with a scalpel.

Discussion Kim and colleagues[58] evaluated the use of selective plantar fasciotomy for forefoot ulcerations in 36 patients and found that 56% of ulcerations healed within 6 weeks. Kitaoka and colleagues[59] evaluated the effect of sectioning the plantar fascia in cadavers and found that after fasciotomy the arch flattened with additional motion in the midfoot and hindfoot joints. To date, little is written about the use of selective plantar fasciotomy and the role it may play in healing of forefoot ulceration. Further research is needed to elicit the effectiveness of this procedure and the potential morbidity associated with it.

Sub–fifth metatarsophalangeal joint (forefoot varus)/styloid process/sub–fifth metatarsal base (forefoot varus)

Introduction Plantar ulcerations occurring on the lateral column may result from relative imbalance or contracture of the tibialis anterior tendon. The tibialis anterior muscle not only functions as a dorsiflexor of the foot but also applies a varus rotation to the foot through its insertions at the medial aspect of the base of the first metatarsal and the medial cuneiform. Lateralization of this tendon through transfer to the lateral cuneiform or cuboid may reduce the deforming force and therefore decrease the lateralized pressures.

Technique A 3-cm incision is made medially at the insertion of the tendon, exposing the tibialis anterior tendon and its sheath. A longitudinal incision is then made through the sheath, allowing visualization of the insertion. The tendon is detached, secured with a whip stitch, and readied for transfer. A tendon passer is used to follow the tendon sheath proximally toward the ankle joint and an incision is made overlying the tendon, exposing it proximally, near the musculotendinous junction. Care is taken to protect the neurovascular bundle that lies lateral to the tendon. The tendon is passed from distal, through the proximal incision. Fluoroscopy is used to visualize the lateral cuneiform and a small incision is made dorsal to the cuneiform. A tendon passer is again used to pass the tendon from the proximal incision through subcutaneous tissues to the lateral aspect of the foot. The foot is held in dorsiflexion and eversion while the tendon is fixated to the cuneiform using an interference screw. This procedure is shown in **Fig. 5**.

Discussion The tibialis anterior tendon transfer, originally described by Garceau[60] and popularized by Ponseti and Campos,[61] is traditionally performed for the management of clubfoot deformity.[60,61] Hoffer and colleagues[62] then described the split tibialis anterior tendon transfer (STATT) as a treatment option for residual clubfoot and spastic equinovarus deformity in adults. Regardless of split or full tendon transfer, the procedures neutralize the varus pull of the tibialis anterior muscle. Henderson and colleagues[63] compared whole tendon transfers and STATTs with regard to plantar pressures after transfer in a cadaveric model. They found that whole and split tendon transfers decreased lateral column pressures overall, with minimal difference in pressure readings between the two.[63] The transfer of the tibialis anterior tendon has sparse literature written about its use in offloading the lateral column in the setting of neuropathic ulcerations, but biomechanically removes a deforming force and balances the foot. Kim and colleagues[64] described a lengthening of the tibialis anterior tendon for lateral column ulcerations; however, long-term results are not yet known.

Plantar central calcaneus (calcaneal gait)

Introduction Ulceration of the plantar heel is most often iatrogenic through overlengthening of the Achilles tendon and creation of a calcaneal gait. As previously described, Achilles tendon lengthening and gastrocnemius recession can be used to treat recalcitrant and nonhealing forefoot ulcerations in the setting of equinus. However, overlengthening of the posterior heel cord can lead to the creation of a calcaneal gait and increased hindfoot pressures during ambulation. The Achilles tendon is overlengthened in 2% to 10% of Achilles lengthening procedures, creating this

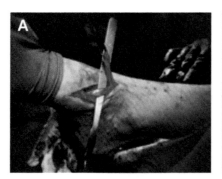
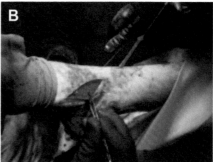
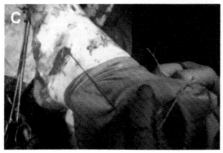

Fig. 5. (A) Detachment of lateral portion of tibialis anterior tendon from insertion for transfer into the cuboid. (B) Lateral portion of STATT (split tibialis anterior tendon transfer) with suture attached. Medial portion shown with forceps remaining attached to the anatomic insertion. (C) Lateral portion of STATT rerouted into the lateral incision and readied for insertion into the cuboid with interference screw. (*Courtesy of* S. Masadeh, DPM, Cincinnati, OH.)

deformity.[47,49,65–67] These ulcerations are often initially treated conservatively through various offloading measures such as bracing, non–weight-bearing, and total contact casting, but remain difficult to manage conservatively. Previously described conservative treatments, such as total contact casting, can have a high rate of complications and a high rate of recurrence because the biomechanical cause of the problem remains uncorrected. Surgical measures are available, and include peroneus brevis transfer, flexor hallucis longus (FHL) transfer with or without calcaneal osteotomy, partial calcanectomy, below-knee amputation, ankle arthrodesis, and tibiotalocalcaneal arthrodesis. Focusing on soft tissue balancing to reduce deformity, this article evaluates the FHL transfer in isolation.

Technique The Achilles tendon paratenon is exposed, which is typically immediately beneath the thin subcutaneous layer. The paratenon is then opened and any pathologic tendon is debrided. Dissection is continued to expose the body of the calcaneus anterior to the insertion of the Achilles tendon, where the FHL tendon is anchored. As dissection continues, the FHL tendon can be visualized, after incising the deep fascia, coursing from lateral to medial within the surgical site. Care must be taken because the neurovascular bundle as well as the FDL course medial to the FHL. The foot is plantarflexed and the FHL tendon is transected as far distal as possible in order to harvest as much length as possible for transfer. The tendon can then be anchored into the calcaneus using a soft tissue anchor or an interference screw. The anchor should be inserted at an angle of 45° in order to maximize pullout strength.[68,69] The surgical site can be closed in a layered anatomic fashion and the foot should be dressed with a dry sterile dressing and splinted in about 10° of plantarflexion, as shown in **Fig. 6**.

Results There is a paucity of literature regarding FHL tendon transfer for the treatment of plantar heel ulcerations after a calcaneal gait. Hahn and colleagues[70] evaluated FHL transfer for the treatment of chronic/neglected Achilles tendon ruptures, with good results noted, as well as a minimal clinical and pedobarographic change in gait pattern in relation to propulsion and the first metatarsophalangeal joint complex. Kim and colleagues[71] retrospectively evaluated 9 patients with diabetes with chronic plantar heel ulcerations caused by calcaneal gait after Achilles tendon overlengthening. All 9 ulcerations healed within 8 weeks after undergoing FHL tendon transfer for treatment.[71]

Discussion Plantar central ulcerations and calcaneal gait are a rare complication of Achilles tendon lengthening, which is likely why there is a lack of research on this topic. There have been several studies suggesting that the FHL is superior to the peroneus brevis for transfer because of superior overall strength of the tendon.[72,73] Most of the literature for tendon transfer procedures for treatment of calcaneal gait is related to acute or recalcitrant Achilles tendon ruptures. More studies are needed to investigate the long-term results regarding rearfoot tendon transfers for the management and treatment of plantar heel ulcerations.

Plantar medial calcaneus (hindfoot valgus)/plantar lateral calcaneus (hindfoot varus)
Introduction Plantar medial and plantar lateral heel ulcerations are commonly cause by a hindfoot valgus or a hindfoot varus foot deformity, respectively. It is important to determine whether the inherent deformity is flexible, semirigid, or a rigid osseous deformity, because this dictates the treatment algorithm. It is also useful to assess relaxed calcaneal stance position (RCSP) and to assess whether this deformity is present throughout the gait cycle.[74] The RCSP is traditionally defined as the angle formed by the bisection of the posterior aspect of the calcaneus and a line drawn perpendicular to the resting surface during relaxed standing in the angle and base of gait, with a value of 0° ± 2° (varus or valgus).[75] Recent literature has raised concerns regarding the basis of RCSP, implying that the original definition of the value of 0° ± 2° by Root and

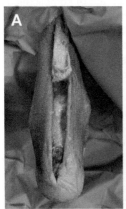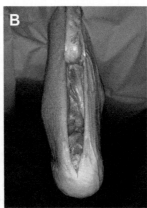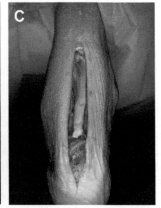

Fig. 6. (*A*) Exposure of the deep fascia deep to the Achilles tendon after transection of the Achilles tendon. (*B*) Exposed FHL tendon readied for harvest and transfer within the deep fascia. (*C*) Transfer of FHL tendon using interference screw at deadman's angle to optimize pullout strength. (*Courtesy of* S. Masadeh, DPM, Cincinnati, OH.)

colleagues[75] has no substantial clinical-based evidence and is merely theoretic. Recent studies have shown that the RCSP is a reliable measure of hindfoot varus and valgus clinically, but challenge the traditional values. These studies have proposed wide-ranging values of 1° varus to 14° valgus in adults, with a mean of 6.07° valgus.[76–78]

Imaging should also be obtained to assess for arthritic changes/rigid deformities, including Harris Beath, calcaneal axial, and hindfoot alignment views to assess the extent of hindfoot varus. In 2010, Lee and colleagues[74] examined the reliability and validity of the commonly used radiographic measurements to diagnose hindfoot varus and valgus. The study determined that naviculocuboid overlap, anteroposterior talonavicular coverage angle, and anteroposterior talus-first metatarsal angle were reliable measurements in distinguishing a hindfoot valgus from varus deformity.[74]

Technique plantar lateral ulcerations

Posterior tibial tendon tenotomy/recession At the medial ankle, just distal to the medial malleolus, a 2-cm incision is made and blunt dissection is performed to the level of the tarsal tunnel. The flexor retinaculum is incised and the posterior tibial tendon is identified. Care is taken not to damage the FDL tendon or the adjacent neurovascular bundle. The tendon is then isolated and either sharply divided or lengthened with a Z-lengthening technique and repaired with nonabsorbable suture, as shown in **Fig. 7**. The surgical site is then closed in a layered anatomic fashion and the foot should be dressed with a dry sterile dressing.[79]

Combined results For hindfoot varus deformities, soft tissue procedures focus on lengthening, transferring, or releasing the overpowering posterior tibial tendon. As described by Huber and colleagues[80] and others, the cavus foot type is driven by agonist/antagonist muscles either by the peroneus longus overpowering the tibialis anterior muscle leading to a plantarflexed first ray (forefoot driven cavus) or the posterior tibial tendon overpowering the peroneus brevis (hindfoot driven varus).[81,82] The decision to lengthen or release versus transfer the posterior tibial tendon has traditionally been determined by whether there is a drop foot or weakness of the anterior compartment causing a steppage gait. Posterior tibial tendon transfers have traditionally been reserved for neurologic or posttraumatic causes (ie, common peroneal nerve injury to increase dorsiflexion strength).[83–85]

For hindfoot valgus deformities, procedures are focused on correcting the overpowering peroneus brevis muscle. The peroneus brevis, as the antagonist to the posterior tibial tendon, pulls the hindfoot into valgus if the posterior tibial tendon is weak. Peroneus brevis tendon lengthening has been described in relation to treating hindfoot valgus in patients with cerebral palsy to reduce deformity.[86]

Discussion It is important when evaluating a hindfoot varus/valgus to clinically assess the biomechanical relationship of the rearfoot to the ground. The authors propose that, in the presence of a wound on either the plantar lateral or plantar medial aspect of the calcaneus, a respective hindfoot varus or hindfoot valgus deformity is the likely cause. Clinical evaluation and judgment, including gait evaluation, and flexibility of deformity, should be used, as opposed to relying on a numerical value. Examining the motion of the hindfoot and reducibility of the deformity is imperative in its correction. A thorough lower extremity examination, including a gait examination, should be included when evaluating patients with hindfoot deformities. Failure to identify proximal deformities, especially with osseous procedures, could increase the potential for failure. Tibia/fibula, knee, hip, and limb length radiographs should be obtained for evaluation.

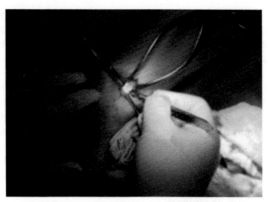

Fig. 7. Posterior tibial tendon is isolated and a Z-lengthening is performed for plantar lateral calcaneus ulcer/hindfoot varus deformity. (*Courtesy of* S. Masadeh, DPM, Cincinnati, OH.)

Because the procedures for hindfoot varus and valgus have only been used in relation to biomechanical deformities and neurologic or posttraumatic causes, further research is required for the use of these procedures in wound healing and ulceration prevention. Long-term studies will also be needed in order to assess for recurrences and efficacy compared with traditional conservative measures.

SUMMARY

Diabetes currently affects approximately 9.4% of the United States population, or roughly 30.3 million citizens.[87] An additional 84.1 million citizens have the diagnosis of prediabetes, a disorder that often progresses to diabetes within 5 years of diagnosis.[87] Because of this, it can be expected that the patient population with diabetes will continue to increase over the next decade, further increasing the medical and economic demands on our society. Between $9 billion and $14 billion dollars was spent directly on the treatment of patients with foot ulcerations in 2015 alone, showing the severe financial implications of foot ulceration.[88,89] Between 15% and 25% of people with diabetes develop a foot ulceration during their lifetimes.[90–92] The estimated cost of treating 1 foot ulcer over a 2-year period is approximately $28,000, with a single hospitalization event exceeding $30,000.[93,94] Given the anticipated increase in the number of patients with diabetes and an annual incidence of ulceration of 2% in those with the diagnosis, it can be safely assumed that the economic burden of ulcerations will continue to increase without establishing more definitive treatment options than the current algorithms offer.[2,94,95]

Knowing that neuropathic ulcerations often progress to the end point of amputations if not treated appropriately in the initial clinic setting, it becomes imperative to treat preulcerative and ulcerative lesions with definitive measures early to save both economic resources and limbs. Ulcerations have been implicated as the causative factor in as many as 84% of amputations in patients with diabetes.[91,96–98] Up to 43% of those patients with diabetes and a foot ulcer progress to an amputation.[98–100] Additional amputations are often inevitable after initial amputation because of the creation of a new deformity and further altering the foot biomechanics and pressure distribution. Reamputation rates have been shown to be as high as 26.7% after 1 year, 48.3% after 3 years, and 60.7% after 5 years, showing the importance of preventing the progression of ulceration and the initial amputation event.[97,101,102]

The typical initial treatment of a diabetic foot ulcer in the clinical setting is often local wound care, offloading through custom orthopedic shoes, or plaster casting to temporarily alleviate the deformity and the increased plantar pressures. These methods have shown efficacy in obtaining initial healing, but reulceration rates remain high. Reulceration rates have been seen as high as 38.8% within 1 year using custom-made footwear and 44.2% with routine care alone, as well as exceeding 60% after 3 years.[4–8] Studies performed by Striesow and colleagues[103] and Viswanathan and colleagues[104] have shown reulceration rates up to 67% in self-selected shoes. Armstrong and colleagues[105] showed an average daily adherence of approximately 28% in those patients with ulceration who were prescribed a removable foot-offloading device, and even the most strictly adherent patients were compliant with their treatment only 60% of the day. Poor outcomes associated with conservative measures are likely caused by persistent hyperglycemia leading to recurrence and poor compliance to the prescribed conservative treatment regimen. This chronic state of increased glucose levels leads to nonenzymatic glycosylation of not only tendons located in the foot and ankle but also throughout the body. Continued protein glycosylation creates contracture, deformity, and imbalance, leading to the creation of high-pressure areas within the weight-bearing surface. To adequately alleviate these increased pressures and reduce the likelihood of recurrence, the source of the deforming force needs to be corrected to regain balance.

Considering the number of current patients with active neuropathic ulceration, it can be assumed that a far greater number are currently in remission, without definitive long-term solution provided. With the greatest risk factor or predictor of ulceration being a prior history of ulceration, it is safe to assume that those patients currently healed will likely reulcerate at a future time.[106] It is therefore imperative to provide longer-lasting, reproducible solutions to address the root of the problem. These solutions can be achieved, in the appropriate situations, through tendon transfer and balancing, not to provide a functional transfer but to reduce the deforming forces creating the deformity itself. These procedures are performed with the intent of restoring a plantigrade, biomechanically neutral foot, improving joint mobility and reducing the associated deformity. The question remains, when should these procedures be performed? It is known that, as a patients continue along the spectrum of ulceration, it likely ends in increasing deformity and amputation. Armstrong and colleagues[105] established a foot surgery classification for patients with diabetes, to stratify risks as (1) elective, (2) prophylactic, (3) curative, or (4) emergent, in nonischemic diabetic patients.[5,107] This hierarchy of surgical classification allows practitioners to readily classify procedures within the patient population with diabetes and predict future outcomes and associated risks with the timing of intervention. This classification was further shown to provide efficacy in treating patients early on the spectrum to prevent progression to eventual amputation, limb loss, or severe postoperative complications.[5,105,107] As the classification level progresses, so does the likelihood of the patient experiencing a poor outcome.[5,105,107] This likelihood further provides support that these patients with ulceration or preulcerative lesions should be treated while in the prophylactic or preulcerative stage when possible, which can often be achieved in flexible or semirigid deformities by removing the deforming forces through the various tendon procedures, based on anatomic ulcer location, as described in this article.

CLINICS CARE POINTS

- Persistent states of hyperglycemia lead to muscular imbalances and the creation of initial flexible deformities.
- Failure to address these deformities leads to biomechanical imbalances and the creation of areas of high pressure on the plantar foot with eventual pursuant ulceration.
- To address these deformities through tendon transfers the deformities must be flexible or semi-rigid.
- Prophylactic surgery may prevent the need for future amputations.

DISCLOSURE

The authors have nothing to disclose.

REFERENCES

1. Apelqvist K, Ragnarson-tennval G, Larsson J, et al. Long term cost for foot ulcers in diabetic patients in a multidisciplinary setting. Foot Ankle Int 1995; 16(7):388–94.
2. Boulton AJ, Vileikyte L, Ragnarson-Tennvall G, et al. The global burden of diabetic foot disease. Lancet 2005;366:719–24.
3. Prompers L, Huijberts M, Schaper N, et al. Resource utilization and costs associated with the treatment of diabetic foot ulcers 2008;51(10):1826–34.
4. Apelqvist J, Larsson J, Agard CD. Long-term prognosis for diabetic patients with foot ulcers. J Intern Med 1993;233:485–91.
5. Armstrong DG, Boulton AJM, Bus SA. Diabetic foot ulcers and their recurrence. N Engl J Med 2017;376(24):2367–75.
6. Bus SA, Waaijman R, Arts M, et al. Effects of custom-made footwear on foot ulcer recurrence in diabetes: a multicenter randomized controlled trial. Diabetes Care 2013;36:4109–16.
7. Laborde JM. Tendon lengthening for neuropathic foot problems. Orthopedics 2010;33(5):319–26.
8. Pound N, Chipchase S, Treece K, et al. Ulcer-free survival following management of foot ulcers in diabetes. Diabet Med 2005;22(10):1306–9.
9. Kearney TP, Hunt NA, Lavery LA. Safety and effectiveness of flexor tenotomies to heal toe ulcers in persons with diabetes. Diabetes Res Clin Pract 2010;89: 224–6.
10. Laborde JM. Neuropathic toe ulcers treated with toe flexor tenotomies. Foot Ankle Int 2007;28(11):1160–4.
11. Rasmussen A, Bjerre-Christensen U, Almdal TP, et al. Percutaneous flexor tenotomy for preventing and treating toe ulcers in people with diabetes mellitus. J Tissue Viability 2013;22:68–73.
12. Schepers T, Berendsen HA, Oei IH, et al. Functional outcome and patient satisfaction after flexor tenotomy for plantar ulcers of the toes. J Foot Ankle Surg 2010;49(2):119–22.
13. Tamir E, McLaren AM, Gadgil A, et al. Outpatient percutaneous flexor tenotomies for management of diabetic claw toe deformities with ulcers: a preliminary report. Can J Surg 2008;51:41–4.
14. Tamir F, Vigler M, Avisar F, et al. Percutaneous tenotomy for the treatment of diabetic toe ulcers. Foot Ankle Int 2014;35:38–43.

15. Van Netten JJ, Bril A, van Baal JG, et al. The effect of flexor tenotomy on healing and prevention of neuropathic diabetic foot ulcers on the distal end of the toe. J Foot Ankle Res 2013;6:3.
16. Bakker K, Apelqvist J, Schaper NC. International working group on diabetic foot editorial board: practical guidelines on the management and prevention of the diabetic foot. Diabetes Metab Res Rev 2013;28:225–31.
17. Hochlenert D, Engels G, Morbach S, et al. Diabetic foot syndrome. Nature. Springer International Publishing AG, Springer; 2018.
18. Cowley MS, Boyko EJ, Shofer JB, et al. Foot ulcer risk and location in relation to prospective clinical assessment of foot shape and mobility among persons with diabetes. Diabetes Res Clin Pract 2008;82:226–32.
19. Thomas R, Brenton K, Harris B, et al. Foot ulceration in a secondary care diabetic clinic population: a 4-year prospective study. Diabetes Res Clin Pract 2010;90:e37–9.
20. Johnson CH, Christensen JC. Biomechanics of the first ray part I. The effects of peroneus longus function: a three-dimensional kinematic study on a cadaver model. J Foot Ankle Surg 1999;38(5):313–21.
21. Berndt AL, Harty M. Transchondral fractures (osteochondritis dissecans) of the talus. J Bone Joint Surg Am 1959;41:988–1020.
22. Glasoe WM, Yack HJ, Saltzman CL. Anatomy and biomechanics of the first ray. Phys Ther 1999;79:854–9.
23. Birke JA, Frankes BD, Foto JG. First ray Joint limitation, pressure, and ulceration of the first metatarsal head in diabetes mellitus. Foot Ankle Int 1995;16(5).
24. Gibbs RC, Boxer MC. Abnormal biomechanics of feet and their cause of hyperkeratosis. J Am Acad Dermatol 1982;6:1061–9.
25. Michaud TM. Foot orthoses and other forms of conservative foot care. Baltimore (MD): Williams & Wilkins; 1993. p. 69–100.
26. Mueller MK, Minor SD, Diamond JE, et al. Relationship of foot deformity to ulcer location in patients with diabetes mellitus. Phys Ther 1990;70:356–62.
27. Roukis TS. Peroneus longus recession. J Foot Ankle Surg 2009;48(3):405–7.
28. DiDomenico LA, AbdelFattah SR, Hassan MK. Emerging concepts with tendon transfers. Podiatry Today 2018. Available at: www.podiatrytoday.com.
29. Dayer R, Assal M. Chronic diabetic ulcers under the first metatarsal head treated by staged tendon balancing: a prospective cohort study. J Bone Joint Surg Br 2009;91(4):487–93.
30. Hamilton GA, Ford LA, Perez H, et al. Salvage of the neuropathic foot by using bone resection and tendon balancing: a retrospective review of 10 patients. J Foot Ankle Surg 2005;44(1):37–43.
31. Birke JA, Sims DS. Plantar sensory thresholds in the insensitive foot. Lepr Rev 1988;10:172–6.
32. Ctercteko GC, Dhanedran M, Hutton WC, et al. Vertical forces acting on the feet of diabetic patients with neuropathic ulceration. Br J Surg 1981;68: 608–14.
33. Cychosz CC, Phisitkul P, Belatti DA, et al. Preventive and therapeutic strategies for diabetic foot ulcers. Foot Ankle Int 2016;37(3):334–43.
34. Grant WP, Sullivan R, Sonenshine DE, et al. Electron microscopic investigation of the effects of diabetes mellitus on the achilles tendon. J Foot Ankle Surg 1997; 36:272–8.
35. Orendurff MS, Rohr ES, Sangeorzan BJ, et al. An equinus deformity of the ankle accounts for only a small amount of the increased forefoot plantar pressure in patients with diabetes. J Bone Joint Surg Br 2006;88:65–8.

36. Couppe C, Svensson RB, Kongsgaard M, et al. Human achilles tendon glycation and function in diabetes. J Appl Physiol 2016;120:130–7.
37. Boulton AJ, Hardisty CA, Betts RP, et al. Dynamic foot pressure and other studies as diagnostic and management aids in diabetic neuropathy. Diabetes Care 1983;6(1):26–33.
38. Frykberg RG, Lavery LA, Pham H, et al. Role of neuropathy and high foot pressures in diabetic foot ulcerations. Diabetes Care 1998;21:1714.
39. Lavery LA, Armstrong DG, Wunderlich RP, et al. Predictive value of foot pressure assessment as part of a population-based diabetes disease management program. Diabetes Care 2003;26(4):1069–73.
40. Veves A, Murray HJ, Young MJ, et al. The risk foot ulceration in diabetic patients with high foot pressure: a prospective study. Diabetologia 1992;35(7): 660–3.
41. Frykberg RG, Bown J, Hall J, et al. Prevalence of equinus in diabetic versus nondiabetic patients. J Am Podiatr Med Assoc 2012;102(2):84–8.
42. Lavery LA, Armstrong DG, Boulton AJ. Diabetes Research Group: ankle equinus deformity and its relationship to high plantar in a large population with diabetes mellitus. J Am Podiatr Med Assoc 2002;92:479.
43. Alazzawi S, Sukeik M, King D, et al. Foot and ankle history and clinical examination: a guide to everyday practice. World J Orthop 2017;18(1):21–9.
44. Barske HL, DiGiovanni BF, Douglass M, et al. Current Concepts Review: isolated gastrocnemius contracture and gastrocnemius recession. Foot Ankle Int 2012; 33(10):915–21.
45. Patel A, DiGiovanni BF. Association between plantar fasciitis and isolated contracture of the gastrocnemius. Foot Ankle Int 2011;32(1):5–8.
46. Colen LB, Kim CJ, Grant WP, et al. Achilles tendon lengthening: friend or foe in the diabetic foot? Plast Reconstr Surg 2013;131:37e–43e.
47. Holstein P, Lohman M, Bitsch M, et al. Achilles tendon lengthening, the panacea for plantar forefoot ulcers? Diabetes Metab Res Rev 2004;20:S37–40.
48. Lin SS, Lee TH, Wapner KL. Plantar forefoot ulceration with equinus deformity of the ankle in diabetic patients; the effect of tendo-achilles lengthening and total contact casting. Orthopedics 1996;19(5):465–75.
49. Mueller MJ, Sinacore DR, Hastings MK, et al. Effect of Achilles tendon lengthening on neuropathic plantar ulcers, a randomized clinical trial. J Bone Joint Surg Am 2003;85-A:1436–45.
50. Cychosz CC, Phisitkul P, Belatti DA, et al. Gastrocnemius recession for foot and ankle conditions in adults: evidence-based recommendations. Foot Ankle Surg 2015;21:77–85.
51. Greenhagen RM, Johnson AR, Peterson MC, et al. Gastrocnemius recession as an alternative to tendoachilles lengthening for relief of forefoot pressure in a patient with peripheral neuropathy: a case report and description of a technical modification. J Foot Ankle Surg 2010;49(2):159.
52. Laborde JM. Neuropathic plantar forefoot ulcers treated with tendon lengthenings. Foot Ankle Int 2008;29(4):378–84.
53. Laborde JM. Midfoot ulcers treated with gastrocnemius soleus recession. Foot Ankle Int 2009;30(9):842–6.
54. Armstrong DG, Stacpoole-Shea S, Nguyen H, et al. Lengthening of the Achilles tendon in diabetic patients who are at high risk for ulceration of the foot. J Bone Joint Surg Am 1999;81(4):535–8.
55. Coughlin MJ, Mann RA. Surgery of the foot and ankle. 7th edition. St Louis (MO): Mosby Inc; 1999.

56. Lippman HI, Perotto A, Farrar R. The neuropathic foot of the diabetic. Bull N Y Acad Med 1976;52(10):1159–78.
57. Ursini F, Arturi F, Nicolosi K, et al. Plantar fascia enthesopathy is highly prevalent in diabetic patients without peripheral neuropathy and correlates with retinopathy and impaired kidney function. PLoS One 2017;12(3): e0174529.
58. Kim JY, Hwang S, Lee Y. Selective plantar fascia release for nonhealing diabetic plantar ulcerations. J Bone Joint Surg Am 2012;94(14):1297–302.
59. Kitaoka HB, Luo ZP, An KN. Effect of plantar fasciotomy on stability of the arch of the foot. Clin Orthop Relat Res 1997;344:307–12.
60. Garceau GJ. Anterior tibial tendon transposition in recurrent congenital club-foot. J Bone Joint Surg Am 1940;22:932–6.
61. Ponseti IV, Campos J. The classic: observations on pathogenesis and treatment of congenital clubfoot. 1972. Clin Orthop Relat Res 2009;467:1124–32.
62. Hoffer MM, Reiswig JA, Garrett AM, et al. The split anterior tibial tendon transfer in the treatment of spastic varus hindfoot of childhood. Orthop Clin North Am 1974;5:31–8.
63. Henderson CP, Parks BG, Guyton GP. Lateral and medial pressures after split versus whole anterior tibialis tendon transfer. Foot Ankle Int 2008;29(10): 1038–41.
64. Kim P, Steinberg J, Kikuchi M, et al. Tibialis anterior tendon lengthening: adjunctive treatment of plantar lateral column diabetic ulcers. J Foot Ankle Surg 2015; 54(4):686–91.
65. Chilvers M, Malicky ES, Anderson JG, et al. Heel overload associated with heel cord insufficiency. Foot Ankle Int 2007;28(6):687–9.
66. Nishimoto GS, Attinger CE, Cooper PS. Lengthening of the Achilles tendon for the treatment of diabetic plantar forefoot ulceration. Surg Clin 2003;83(3): 707–26.
67. Schweinberger MH, Roukis TS. Surgical correction of soft-tissue ankle equinus contracture. Clin Podiatr Med Surg 2008;25(4):571–85.
68. Burkhart SS, Lo IKY, Brady PC. Burkhart's view of the shoulder: a cowboy's guide to advanced shoulder arthroscopy. Philadelphia: Lippincott Williams & Wilkins; 2006.
69. Strauss E, Frank D, Kubiak E, et al. The effect of the ankle of suture anchor insertion on fixation failure at the tendon-suture interface after rotator cuff repair: deadman's angle revisited. Arthroscopy 2009;25:597.
70. Hahn F, Maiwald C, Horstmann T, et al. Changes in plantar pressure distribution after achilles tendon augmentation with flexor hallucis longus transfer. Clin Biomech (Bristol, Avon) 2008;23(1):109–16.
71. Kim J-Y, Lee I, Seo K, et al. FHL tendon transfer in diabetics for treatment of non-healing plantar heel ulcers. Foot Ankle Int 2010;31(6):480–5.
72. Sebastian H, Datta B, Maffulli N, et al. Mechanical properties of reconstructed Achilles tendon with transfer of peroneus brevis or flexor hallucis longus tendon. J Foot Ankle Surg 2007;46(6):424–8.
73. Silver RL, de la Garza K, Rang M. The myth of muscle balance: a study of relative strengths and excursions of normal muscles about the foot and ankle. J Bone Joint Surg Br 1985;67:432–7.
74. Lee KM, Chung CY, Park MS, et al. Reliability and validity of radiographic measurements in hindfoot varus and valgus. J Bone Joint Surg Am 2010;92(13): 2319–27.

75. Root ML, Orien WP, Weed JH. Biomechanical examination of the foot. Los Angeles (CA): Clinical Biomechanics corp; 1971.
76. Payne C, Richardson M. Changes in measurement of neutral and relaxed calcaneal stance positions with experience. Foot 2000;10(2):81–3.
77. Sobel E, Levitz SJ, Caselli MA, et al. Reevaluation of the relaxed calcaneal stance position. Reliability and normal values in children and adults. J Am Podiatr Med Assoc 1999;89(5):258–64.
78. Weiner-Oglivie S, Rome K. The reliability of three techniques for measuring foot position. J Am Podiatr Med Assoc 1998;88(8):381–6.
79. Redfern JC, Thordarson DB. Achilles lengthening/posterior tibial tenotomy with immediate weightbearing for patients with significant comorbidities. Foot Ankle Int 2008;29(3):325–8.
80. Huber M. What is the role of tendon transfer in the cavus foot. Foot Ankle Clin 2013;18(4):689–95.
81. Chilvers M, Manoli A. The subtle cavus foot and association with ankle instability and lateral foot overload. Foot Ankle Clin 2008;13(2):315–24.
82. Rosenbaum AJ, Lisella J, Patel N, et al. The cavus foot. Med Clin 2014;98(2): 301–12.
83. Mayer L. The physiologic method of tendon transplantation in the treatment of paralytic drop-foot. J Bone Joint Surg Am 1937;19(2):389–94.
84. Richardson DR, Nathan LG. The bridle procedure. Foot Ankle Clin 2011;16(3): 419–33.
85. Rodriguez RP. The bridle procedure in the treatment of paralysis of the foot. Foot Ankle 1992;13(2):63–9.
86. Nather A, Bee CD, Huak CY, et al. Epidemiology of diabetic foot problems and predictive factors for limb. J Diabetes Complications 2008;22:77–82.
87. Centers for Disease Control and Prevention. National diabetes statistics report. Atlanta (GA): Centers for Disease Control and Prevention, U.S. Department of Health and Human Services; 2017.
88. Rice JB, Desai U, Cummings AK, et al. Burden of diabetic foot ulcers for medicare and private insurers. Diabetes Care 2014;37(3):651–8.
89. Singer AJ, Tassiopoulos A, Kirsner RS. Evaluation and management of lower extremity ulcers. N Engl J Med 2017;377:1559–67.
90. Bakker K, Haper NS. The development of global consensus guidelines on the management and prevention of the diabetic foot 2011. Diabetes Metab Res Rev 2012;28:116–8.
91. Pecoraro RE, Reiber GE, Burgess EM. Pathways to diabetic limb amputation. Basis for prevention. Diabetes Care 1990;13:513–21.
92. Singh N, Armstrong DG, Lipsky BA. Preventing foot ulcers in patients with diabetes. J Am Med Assoc 2005;293:217–28.
93. Hicks CW, Selvarajah S, Mathiodoudakis N, et al. Trends and determinants of costs associated with the inpatient care of diabetic foot ulcers. J Vasc Surg 2014;60(5):1247–54.
94. Ramsey SD, Newton K, Blough D, et al. Incidence outcomes and costs of foot ulcers in patients with diabetes. Diabetes Care 1999;22:382–7.
95. Schaper NC, Van Netten JJ, Apelqvist J, et al. Prevention and management of foot problems in diabetes: a summary guidance for daily practice based on the 2015 IWGDF guidance documents. Diabetes Metab Res Rev 2016. https://doi.org/10.1002/dmrr.2695.
96. Frykberg RG, Zgonis T, Armstrong DG, et al. Diabetic foot disorders: a clinical practice guideline. J Foot Ankle Surg 2006;45:S1–66.

97. Larsson J, Agardh CD, Apelqvist J, et al. Long-term prognosis after healed amputation in patients with diabetes. Clin Orthop Relat Res 1998;350:149–58.

98. Moss SE, Klein BE. Long-term incidence of lower-extremity amputation in a diabetic population. Arch Fam Med 1996;5:391–8.

99. Connel FA, Shaw C, Will J. Lower extremity amputations among persons with diabetes mellitus. Morb Mortal Wkly Rep 1991;40:737–9.

100. Reiber GE, Boyko EJ, Smith DG. Lower extremity foot ulcers and amputations in diabetes. In: Harris MI, Cowie C, Stern MP, editors. Diabetes in America. 2nd edition. Bethesda (MD): National Institutes of Health; 1995. p. 409–28.

101. Chu YJ, Li XW, Wang PH, et al. Clinical outcomes of toe amputation in patients with type 2 diabetes in Tianjin, China. Int Wound J 2016;13(2):175–81.

102. Izumi Y, Satterfield K, Lee S, et al. Risk of reamputation in diabetic patients stratified by limb and level of amputation: a 10-year observation. Diabetes Care 2006;29(3):566–70.

103. Striesow F. Special manufactured shoes for prevention of recurrent ulcer in diabetic foot syndrome. Med Klin 1998;93(12):695–700.

104. Viswanathan V, Madhavan S, Gnanasundaram S, et al. Effectiveness of different types of footwear insoles for the diabetic neuropathic foot. Diabetes Care 2004; 27:474–7.

105. Armstrong DG, Lavery LA, Kimbriel HR, et al. Activity patterns of patients with diabetic foot ulceration. Diabetes Care 2003;26(9):2595–997.

106. Monteiro-Soares M, Boyko EJ, Ribeiro J, et al. Predictive factors for diabetic foot ulceration: a systematic review. Diabetes Metab Res Rev 2012;28:574–600.

107. Armstrong DG, Frykberg RG. Classifying diabetic foot surgery: toward a rational definition. Diabet Med 2003;20:329–31.

A Novel Limb Salvage Technique of External Fixation Protection of Lower Extremity Plastic Reconstructions with Immediate Postoperative Ambulation (Bibbo Flap and Frame Technique)

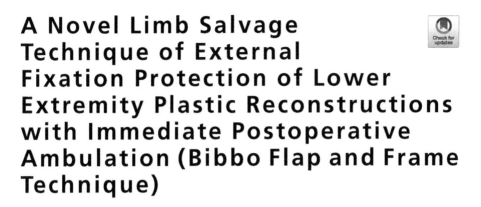

Christopher Bibbo, DO, DPM

KEYWORDS

- Bibbo flap & frame technique • Lower extemity plastic reconstruction
- Post-operative ambulation • Amputations • External fixation

KEY POINTS

- Non–weight bearing is mandatory after soft tissue reconstructions of the weight-bearing and the high-pressure areas in the lower extremity.
- The typical external fixator constructs used for this technique are circular external fixators with fine wires (half-pins are optional).
- Plastic reconstructions within each zone of the lower extremity have requisite characteristics particular to a region, which must be incorporated into the ExFix design.
- The levels of amputation indicated for external fixation for immediate postoperative ambulation include the ankle level (Syme), below-knee amputation, above-knee amputation, and hip disarticulation.

INTRODUCTION

Non–weight bearing is mandatory after soft tissue (ST) reconstructions of the weight-bearing and the high-pressure areas in the lower extremity. The most common method of patient mobilization after surgical reconstruction of chronic foot and ankle wounds has been to place patients non–weight bearing with crutches, walkers, or a

Foot & Ankle Surgery, Plastic Reconstructive & Microsurgery, Orthopaedic Trauma and MSK Infection Services, Rubin Institute for Advanced Orthopaedics, International Center for Limb Lengthening, Sinai Hospital of Baltimore, 2401 West Belvedere Avenue, Baltimore, MD 21215, USA
E-mail address: drchrisbibbo@gmail.com

Clin Podiatr Med Surg 38 (2021) 55–71
https://doi.org/10.1016/j.cpm.2020.09.003
0891-8422/21/© 2020 Elsevier Inc. All rights reserved.

wheelchair. Often patients are older, have more complex medical comorbidities, are deconditioned, and simply cannot comply with the prescribed weight-bearing status with these methods, which leads to deconditioning, depression, or noncompliance. Noncompliance quickly leads to failure of the reconstructive effort and the serious threat of limb loss. Limited mobility also may lead to social isolation, which may result in ignored medical problems, repeat hospitalization, social isolation, and depression. Thus, the most common methods of protecting the reconstructive site (and amputation site) and patient mobilization are difficult for many patients, with many resorting to noncompliance, putting the patient at significant jeopardy for major morbidity. These issues also contribute to longer hospital and rehabilitation facility lengths of stay and increased health care costs.

The use of external fixation (ExFix) for wound stabilization was described by Bibbo in 2006.[1] Inspired by the concept of ExFix and wound management in respect to previously described limitations of postoperative care after ST reconstructions, the idea of incorporating the inherent advantages of immediate mobilization and the potential for immediate ambulation gained with ExFix, the use of ExFix to also protect ST reconstruction of wounds, flaps, and skin grafts was realized. In 2008, Bibbo performed first performed circular ring ExFix for ST protection with weight-bearing mobilization in a noncompliant patient with a neglected calcaneus gait, possessing a relatively smaller plantar heel wound and calcaneal osteomyelitis. The index surgery of tendon transfers with local ST rearrangement was met on postoperative day 1 by unauthorized patient weight bearing, resulting in loss of the reconstructive effort, a worsened wound, and further exposure of the calcaneus. A second surgery of radical débridement, reverse sural flap, and placement of an ExFix subsequently was performed, salvaging the limb (**Fig. 1**). Over the course of 19 years, the author has performed several hundred various ST (and bone) reconstructions of the lower extremity in conjunction with ExFix to provide protective off-loading of ST reconstructions, allow access for any type of wound care, monitor the reconstruction, and allow immediate weight-bearing mobilization (**Table 1**); even simultaneous bilateral reconstructions have been managed in this manner (**Fig. 2**). The vast experience of the author has allowed for refinement of his technique from the inception to the current state of the art. Colloquially, the

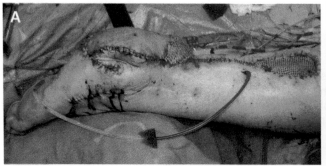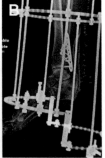

Fig. 1. (*A*) Reverse sural flap combined with ExFix (2008) for plantar heel defect with osteomyelitis after premature, unauthorized weight bearing after an index surgery for a lesser heel wound. This was the original case for the F&F technique. Note the flap is inset with the foot on plantar-flexion to extend the reach of the flap. (*B*) Radiograph (2008) of the off-loading ExFix used to float the heel of the flap shown in Fig. 1A off any surface ground during healing while allowing partial weight bearing. (With Permission. Copyright 2020, Dr. Christopher Bibbo Main Street Enterprises, LLC, DBA Global Medicus.)

Table 1
List of flap and soft tissue reconstructions combined with external fixation off-loading the author has performed

Anatomic Site	Flap Reconstruction	External Fixation Function	External Fixation Construct
Forefoot	V-Y and abductor hallucis flaps; large skin grafts, wound care, NPWD	Off-loading and ambulation	Circular fine wire
Midfoot	V-Y, intrinsic muscle flaps; skin grafts, wound care and NPWD; large skin grafts	Off-loading; ambulation	Circular fine wire
Plantar foot (especially calcaneus)	PMA flap alone, or in combination with intrinsic muscle flaps; large skin grafts; wound care and NPWB; neurovascular repairs with trauma	Off-load; ambulation; immobilize joint during healing	Circular fine wire
Plantar-posterior heel junction	Reverse sural + PMA, reduction calcaneoplasty ± foot flaps; skin grafts; wound care and NPWD	Off-load; ambulation; equinus position to extend reach of reverse sural flap; facilitate local wound care	Circular fine wire Equinus frame as needed
Ankle	Reverse peroneus brevis; reverse hemisoleus; reverse sural; extensor digitorum brevis; PMA flap, distally based vascularized fibula flap; propeller flaps; skin grafts; ExFix-assisted wound closure; neurovascular repairs, wound care and NPWD	Immobilize joint during healing; ambulate; off-load posterior, lateral, medial ankle; facilitate local wound care	Circular fine wire Equinus frame as needed Transarticular pin-bar
Posterior heel	Reverse hemisoleus, reverse sural, reverse peroneus brevis w/ without bone or skin, reverse flexor hallucis muscle flaps; reduction osteoplasty; wound care, NPWD	Ambulate; off-load; immobilize joint during healing; facilitate local wound care	Circular fine wire Equinus frame as needed

(continued on next page)

Table 1
(continued)

Anatomic Site	Flap, Reconstruction	External Fixation Function	External Fixation Construct
Posterior leg	Local skin flaps; skin grafts; ExFix-assisted wound closure; wound care and NPWD	Off-loading; facilitate local wound care	Circular fine wire Equinus frame as needed
Leg	Free fibula; latissimus major free flap; ALT free flap; reverse sural, combined gastrocnemius, soleus flaps, toe flexor flaps; wound care and NPWD; ExFix-assisted wound closure	Offloading; facilitate local wound care; restrict joint ROM	Circular fine wire
Pelvis	Biceps femoris flap; wound care and NPWD	Stabilization for healing; off-loading adjunct; facilitate local wound care	Pin-bar
Elbow	Flexor carpi ulnaris flap; lateral arm flap; local fasciocutaneous flaps; full-thickness skin grafts; traumatic tissue injury; local wound care and NPWD	Offload pressure; immobilize Joint for flap healing; facilitate local wound care; restrict joint ROM	Circular fine wire in extension Unilateral pin-bar
Hand and wrist	Intrinsic hand muscle and carpal flaps; wound care and NPWD	Immobilize joint for healing; off-load	Unilateral pin-bar and circular fine wire

Abbreviations: ALT, anterolateral thigh free flap; NPWD, negative pressure wound dressing.

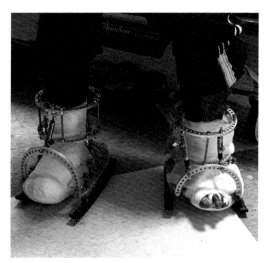

Fig. 2. Bilateral F&F for a patient who underwent simultaneous PMA flaps for a plantar heel ST defect with calcaneal osteomyelitis. The patient performed immediate weight bearing, able to ambulate with a walker at hospital discharge to home. (With Permission. Copyright 2020, Dr. Christopher Bibbo Main Street Enterprises, LLC, DBA Global Medicus.)

concept of using an ExFix to protect an ST/bone reconstruction while mobilizing the patient is referred to the Bibbo flap and frame (F&F) technique, with *flap* referring to any ST reconstruction and *frame* referring to the ExFix. Additionally, Bibbo adapted his concept to the protection of primary amputation sites, and revision amputations with ST reconstructions, for below-knee, above-knee, and hip-level amputations. Bibbo's technique ExFix coupled with an immediate postoperative prosthesis (IPOP) allows protection of the amputation site (primary or revision) protection, edema control, and immediate full weight-bearing ambulation until a permanent prosthesis is fitted.[2] This strategy has radically improved the postoperative rehabilitation of patients with major lower extremity amputations as well enhanced these patients' ability to resume their lives in the postoperative period. This novel IPOP coupled to a ring ExFix now is available commercially as the X-Prosthesis (Post-Op Innovations, Fallston, Maryland).

CONSTRUCTING THE EXTERNAL FIXATOR FOR THE FLAP AND FRAME TECHNIQUE

The typical ExFix constructs used for this technique are circular ExFix with fine wires (half-pins are optional). The ExFix is constructed to allow immediate progressive weight bearing while protecting the healing of wound reconstruction. Additionally, if deformity correction is desired at the same time, the ExFix may incorporate all or part of a 6-axis deformity correction system. The use of the ExFix for ST protection with immediate ambulation essentially has been a game changer in the surgical management of lower extremity wound throughout the perioperative period (and, in a slightly different fashion, the upper extremity).

Key components for the F&F technique are choice of ExFix components (**Box 1**) and the configuration of the ExFix. Often, F&F technique patients may be deconditioned and weak, possess multiple medical comorbidities, and have limited abilities to complete activities of daily living without the ability to ambulate. These issues must be

---

Box 1
Essential external fixation components required for the flap and frame technique

Skinny wires: smooth and olive

Half-pins (optional)

Circular rings: all sizes—larger than normal use

Half-rings: to create reverse rocker stabilization platform

Threaded rods: all sizes

Fast adjusting struts (TrueLok): all sizes, multiple back-up parts

Hexapod rings and struts, e-Tabs (Hexapod): for deformity correction

Walking rockers

Postoperative shoe/cast boot: to create a sole for external fixator

---

addressed by the use of a lightweight, durable device that has a proved track record. Additionally, modularity is a desired feature, because a temporary ExFix can be modified into a weight-bearing construct. In the remote past, the author used carbon fiber rings and associated components but found that unreliability resulted in multiple ExFix revision. The author has found that use of aluminum alloy rings and compatible componentry, features of modularity, capability of performing acute adjustments with struts, and 6-axis mounting capabilities with user-friendly, powerful software programming meet all the hardware needs to perform an F&F procedure. The author has found the ExFix system unsurpassed in providing all these features are the True-Lok and Hexapod systems (Orthofix, Lewisville, Texas).

EXTERNAL FIXATOR CONSTRUCT SPECIFICATIONS BY LOWER EXTREMITY ZONE

Plastic reconstructions within each zone of the lower extremity have requisite characteristics particular to a region, which must be incorporated into the ExFix design. The surgeon must know, however, that, unlike circular ExFix's for relatively heathy patients undergoing typical deformity or bone corrections, modifications must be made to the ExFix in most all F&F cases. Unlike rings that are as close as possible to the limb in healthy patients, ring sizes must be increased. This concept of expanded ring size is to provide extra room to off-load and protect the reconstruction but also allow wound care, easy visualization, obesity, and accommodating massive fluctuating edema (**Fig. 3**). Densely neuropathic patients have a poorly expounded propensity for tibial shaft fractures associated with half-pin fixation of the tibial shaft. In metaphyseal bone, these patients seem to do well with half-pins. Thus, Ilizarov wires (skinny wires or fine wires) should be used on multiple, if not all, rings. Usually, by virtue of the needs of the reconstructive effort, rings bordering and within the level of the plastic reconstruction are spaced farther apart than normal; this construct may need to be revised in a modular fashion. Finally, the ExFix configuration must be constructed to allow immediate or graduated weight bearing, keeping in mind both knee and hip mechanics. The plantar foot is the region originally described by Bibbo for the F&F technique, and remains the most common location for protected ambulation (see **Fig. 1**). The other zones are the posterior heel, posterior leg, posterior-plantar heel junction, forefoot/midfoot, and expanded ankle region.

Plantar heel coverage frequently is covered by the specialized tissue of the plantar medial artery (PMA) flap for reconstructions of infections, trauma, and even tumors.[3]

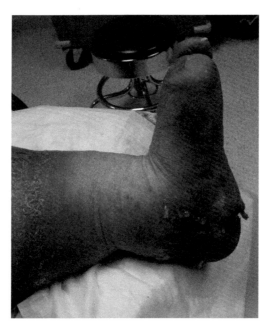

Fig. 3. Necrotic diabetic heel ulcer with calcaneal osteomyelitis. This patient has a massive body habitus with acute on chronic high-volume fluctuating edema. In this patient population, the need for larger than usual ring sizes and an extremely stable ExFix construct cannot be overemphasized. (With Permission. Copyright 2020, Dr. Christopher Bibbo Main Street Enterprises, LLC, DBA Global Medicus.)

Because flaps provide fill and resurfacing, the PMA flap often is supplemented by intrinsic muscle filler flaps. The donor site is managed with a skin graft with or without a neodermal in-growth matrix. A free flap, such as the anterolateral thigh, rectus, latissimus dorsi, or gracilis flap, also may be used. Both the flap and donor sites must be assured to be floated off the ground—this is not negotiable. Often it takes 2 months to 3 months for the flap to appropriately heal, to allow weight-bearing pressure on the ST reconstruction. Generally, a 2-ring tibial block and a footplate with skinny wires in the rearfoot/midfoot/forefoot, based on the availability a placement site, that does not violate the ST reconstruction. Quick-adjust struts are used, allowing easy access and custom positioning of the foot during surgery. Typically, the ExFix is placed after the ST reconstruction, but, in large patients, placement of the proximal rings may assist during the case, acting to elevate the limb (**Fig. 4**). Rockers, or a dummy ring, are placed below the foot ring. It is critical to accurately assess adequate offloading depth protection from the ground and any possible environmental objects. Placing a threaded rod on the across the dummy ring may be helpful to provide additional protection of the plantar surface of the foot. A note of caution is that rockers add weight to an ExFix and may cause a posterior knee thrust during gait (dynamic genu recurvatum) in patients with weakened quadriceps and hamstrings. A plantar walking sole created by using the bottom of a cast shoe attached to the foot or dummy ring is a lightweight device that provides traction and a wide area of protection.

The posterior heel frequently is covered by the reverse sural flap and distally based muscle flaps: reverse hemisoleus, flexor halluces longus, peroneus brevis. Free flaps used to cover the plantar foot also frequently are used to cover this zone (discussed

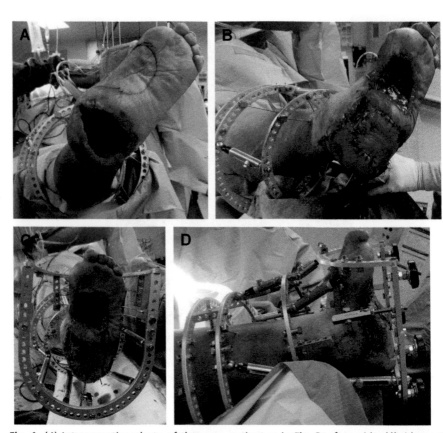

Fig. 4. (*A*) Intraoperative photo of the same patient as in **Fig. 3**, after wide débridement. Note that the proximal tibial block rings were placed first, acting as leg holders to elevate the limb. The extrawide ring size is readily apparent. (*B*) Defect filled with intrinsic muscle turnover flaps followed by a planter medial artery flap. Donor site and non–weight-bearing gap covered with neodermal ingrowth matrix. Note the use of a drain-mitigation of hematoma formation is critical. Note the use of 3 very wide tibial rings to accommodate patient size and high-volume fluctuating edema. Rapid adjust struts (TrueLok) are used to allow immediate acute custom positioning of the extremity and facilitate perioperative ST care. (*C*) Plantar view highlighting the wide rings and foot plate, and multiple rapid adjustable struts. An optional half-pin is placed in the calcaneus in very large patients to assist in maintaining foot position. (*D*) Lateral view intraoperative of completed F&F technique. Prior to the development of walking rockers, walking legs made from table leg components were placed on the foot ring (2012) to float the flap off the ground during ambulation. (With Permission. Copyright 2020, Dr. Christopher Bibbo Main Street Enterprises, LLC, DBA Global Medicus.)

previouslyd). The F&F ExFix that protects this region follows the same principles, described previously, for the plantar zone. Additionally, the foot and tibial rings must be shifted more posterior to allow a wide space between the posterior heel (flap site) and the posterior leg (flap donor site). Fast adjust struts are placed strategically to allow accommodate patient supine positioning in bed, prevent objects protruding on the STs, and allow unfettered access while maintaining ExFix stability when 1 strut or 2 struts are retracted from position during ST care. When long fast struts are long, the author ensures that struts are placed as close as possible to the sagittal plane to counter the concentration of forces that occur at this site (**Fig. 5**).

The posterior/plantar heel junction is a special area that may be covered by a combination of the PMA and reverse sural flaps or distally based muscle flaps. Both flaps as well as the flap donor sites must be protected. When reach of any flap covering this zone is pushed to the limit and coverage is shy of the goal, placing the ExFix in plantar flexion (equinus frame) helps the flaps the distant extend of coverage needed (**Fig. 6**). When a free flap anastomosis is off the posterior tibial vessels, mild plantar flexion of 3° to 5° can relax and protect the microanastomosis suture line. When the ST reconstruction is well healed, the ExFix may be brought gradually to a neutral position. The concept of placing a limb in plantar flexion also is applied for reduction osteoplasty.[4]

The posterior leg often is a site for donor site reconstruction, skin grafts, negative pressure wound dressings, and flaps. Pressure relief is used most often when a patient is supine in bed or in various forms of chair sitting; off-loading this region may be focal or expansive (**Fig. 7**). Reverse rockers are applied when the span is wide, stabilizing the limb and providing extra height (see **Fig. 7**). When the ST reconstruction is intimate with other anatomic structures that cross the ankle, however, then ankle stability is mandatory. Similarly, the anterior, lateral, and medial lower extremity ST

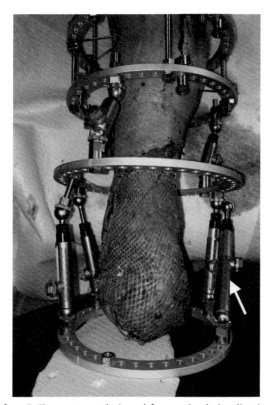

Fig. 5. Example of an ExFix construct designed for maximal visualization of the ST reconstruction while allowing active ankle motion and full weight-bearing ambulation. Note the rapid adjust struts are placed such that when one is detached (*arrow*), the stability of the ExFix is not violated. (With Permission. Copyright 2020, Dr. Christopher Bibbo Main Street Enterprises, LLC, DBA Global Medicus.)

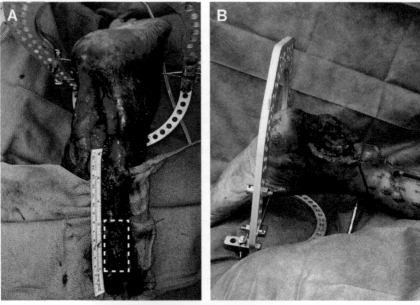

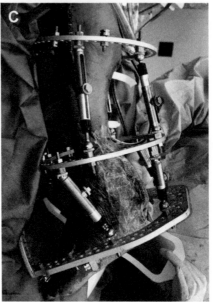

Fig. 6. (*A*) Diabetic posterior distal leg/ankle/heel wound with osteomyelitis managed by reverse flexor hallucis longus myo-osseous flap: the vascularized fibula component of the flap (outlined [*dashed lines*]) is contained within the flexor hallucis longus muscle, fed by the retrograde flow of the distal peroneal perforators via the distal arterial circuit. Note the foot assembly with large foot ring, allowing ample posterior off-loading, also assisting to elevate the foot. (*B*) Lateral view of myo-osseous flap inset with foot in plantar-flexed position. An off-loading equinus frame for ambulation is ideal to relax the flap. (*C*) Intraoperative photo of myo-osseous flap to calcaneus/ankle after F&F technique. Note: equinus position, selection of patient to weight bear of forefoot, use of rapid adjust struts, oversized rings for ST care/negative pressure wound dressing changes, and use only of Ilizarov skinny wires. (With Permission. Copyright 2020, Dr. Christopher Bibbo Main Street Enterprises, LLC, DBA Global Medicus.)

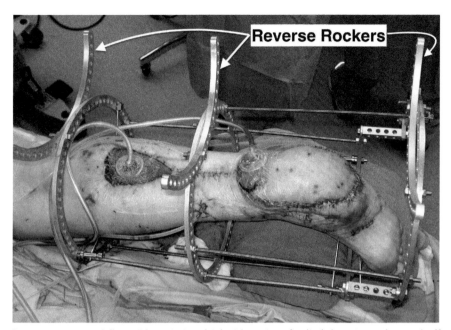

Fig. 7. Reverse sural flap with ExFix in a high-risk patient for limb loss. Note the total off-loading of posterior leg/ankle with widely spanned frame and reverse rockers that help with stability and elevation in bed; the foot is in slight equinus to facilitate additional distal reach of the flap onto the planter surface of the foot. The foot is off-loaded for guided ambulation. The basic configuration of this ExFix allows for modularity, and can be modified as needed. (With Permission. Copyright 2020, Dr. Christopher Bibbo Main Street Enterprises, LLC, DBA Global Medicus.)

reconstructions may require off-loading protection. When a flap or other ST reconstruction crosses the ankle, limited or zero range of motion (ROM) is desired; the ExFix is locked statically, or in mild plantarflexion, as described previously. Examples are a propeller flap covering the anterior and medial ankle (**Fig. 8**) and the reverse peroneus brevis muscle flap or flexor halluces longus myo-osseous flap (muscle + fibula bone) to cover the lateral ankle and calcaneus, respectively (see **Fig. 6**).

Deformity correction by distraction osteogenesis, compression arthrodesis, or angular correction may be executed simultaneously with the F&F technique.[5–7] The section of ExFix that addresses area involved with the deformity correction is constructed in true fashion for the deformity correction execution while the off-loaded area may be modified to satisfy off-loading (**Fig. 9**). Because weight bearing may be limited during deformity correction, if weight bearing is necessary, the deformity correction site sometimes may be sequestered within an overriding mother frame, an example of the ship in a bottle technique.

The F&F technique is such a powerful technique that the author has applied the concept to ExFix-assisted wound closure[8] (**Fig. 10**) and the upper extremity. The F&F approach is applicable to ST coverage needs of the wrist, hand, and elbow. The elbow is especially prone to pressure and shear forces, and strict attention to off-loading and restricted elbow ROM may be achieved by F&F technique (**Fig. 11**). **Table 1** lists of various uses ExFix for ST reconstructions used by the author.

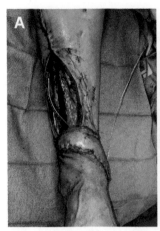
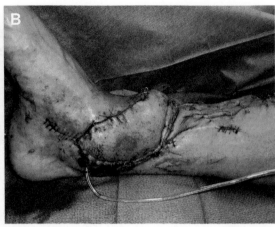

Fig. 8. Anterior view (*A*) and medial view (*B*) of a propeller flap to cover the anterior and medial ankle. Restricted motion is desired for flaps crossing the ankle in any plane, relaxing the vascular pedicle and suture line, thus promoting more rapid healing and ultimately a stable ST reconstruction. (With Permission. Copyright 2020, Dr. Christopher Bibbo Main Street Enterprises, LLC, DBA Global Medicus.)

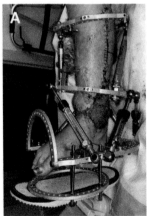
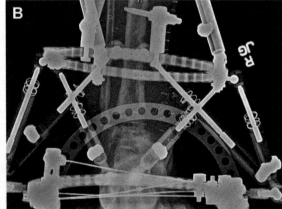

Fig. 9. Photo (*A*) and radiograph (*B*) of patient with tibial bone loss and ankle wound after partial necrosis of a propeller flap, then supplemented with a reverse hemisoleus flap and skin graft. The frame stabilizes and protects the flaps while continuing active 6-axis correction for varus and compression arthrodesis (*B*). Note: programmed deformity correction struts between wide accommodative tibia-foot rings (Hexapod), Ilizarov skinny wires, frame extension to accommodate limb length discrepancy (prior to proximal distraction osteogenesis), and traction walking sole. (With Permission. Copyright 2020, Dr. Christopher Bibbo Main Street Enterprises, LLC, DBA Global Medicus.)

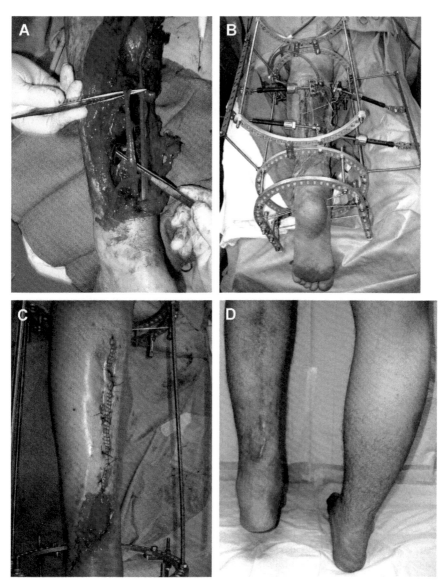

Fig. 10. Agriculture injury with exposed vital structures (*A*). ExFix driven wound closure (*B*); note the specialized frame with a wide area for active mechanical wound care while allowing partial weight-bearing ambulation. Wound at the end of ExFix wound closure (*C*). Final reconstructive result (*D*); note the ability to achieve heel lift. (With Permission. Copyright 2020, Dr. Christopher Bibbo Main Street Enterprises, LLC, DBA Global Medicus.)

AMPUTATIONS AND EXTERNAL FIXATION

The levels of amputation indicated for ExFix for immediate postoperative ambulation include the ankle-level (Syme) amputation, below-knee amputation, above-knee amputation, and hip disarticulation. By virtue of the very short loss of limb length with the Syme amputation, the off-loading of the Syme ST calcaneal/heel flap and

A   B   C

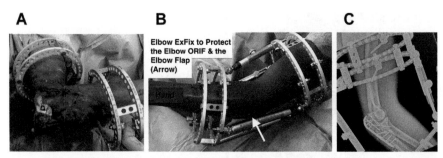

Elbow ExFix to Protect
the Elbow ORIF & the
Elbow Flap
(Arrow)

Fig. 11. F&F technique applied to the upper extremity. Farming injuring with open olecranon fracture; proximal and distal rings applied after open reduction and internal fixation (*A*). Final frame construct (*B*) applied in extension to protect the elbow flap (*arrow*) and the internal fixation of the fracture (*C*). (With Permission. Copyright 2020, Dr. Christopher Bibbo Main Street Enterprises, LLC, DBA Global Medicus.)

associated tendon transfers is addressed the standard F&F technique with a circular fine wire or hybrid construct.[9] After major lower extremity amputations (below-knee amputations, above-knee amputations, and hip disarticulations), patients have been restricted to a non–weight-bearing status of the operative limb, achieved in a wheelchair or bed; only a very well-conditioned patient achieves non–weight bearing on the amputated limb with a walker. Patients undergoing major amputations often have fragile STs. Moreover, patients undergoing revision amputation require combinations of muscle flaps, skin grafts, and negative pressure wound dressing; all of these are vital to assist in maintaining the level of amputation in revision surgery.[10,11] The traditional IPOP as well as other commercially available IPOPs (which are not placed immediately; they are placed in a delayed manner) are unsuitable for use unless the patient is a healthy young patient with a near normal ST envelope; this patient is in the minority of patients undergoing lower extremity amputation. Additionally, these IPOPs do not allow for immediate ambulation on a residual limb with healing STs, nor allow for continued wound care.

A novel IPOP, the X-Prosthesis, recently has come on the market (**Fig. 12**A). The X-Prosthesis mitigates all of down-sides of traditional IPOPs, allowing immediate ambulation on fresh amputations, especially those amputations with associated complex ST reconstructions and wound care needs. The author's data continue to show that the X-Prosthesis allows immediate ambulation on the amputated extremity, prevents physical deconditioning, improves hospital depression scores, decreases the hospital/rehabilitation facility length of stay, and promotes an earlier return to independent home living and social mainstreaming. The X-Prosthesis has shown a major positive on ambulation potential and permanent prosthetic fitting. The author's data also demonstrated the positive effect of elevating Medicare Functional Level, K-level walking status: unilateral wheelchair bound amputees (K-0) have risen to home ambulation amputee patients (K-2) or limited community ambulators (K-3). Likewise, previous K-1 and K-2 ambulators have risen to the functional level of being independent societal walkers (K-3). Placement of the permanent prosthesis has improved to a time of as little as 2 months, compared with 6 months to 8 months in high-risk patients.

Simply, the amputation is performed per surgeon technique, including any ST procedures or application of any associated wound care devices. Below-knee amputations are addressed by placing either a below-knee circular ExFix, or at least 2

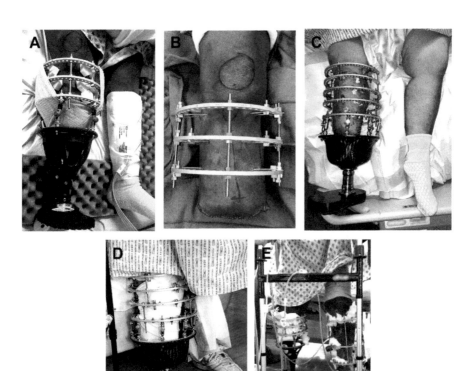

Fig. 12. (*A*) The X-Prosthesis. Note: adjustable pilon, foot plate, and apertures for wound care and drainage of fluids. The X-Prosthesis can be removed from the ExFix by a rapid release mechanism. This typically is placed in the recovery room and immediate limb motion commenced. Ambulation has been as early in the recovery room. (*B*) Ilizarov wires and wider rings for edema are used for the X-Prosthesis. When the ExFix block must be placed very proximal, the proximal ring may be a half or three-quarter ring to accommodate knee flexion. (*C, D*) X-Prosthesis patient with a low below-knee amputation, which conserves oxygen consumption during gait, decreases final prosthetic weight, and improves the fit of the final prosthesis (*C*). This 525-lb patient required multiple rings placed with a hybrid fixation technique. This patient is shown standing postoperative day 1, beginning gait training with a walker (*D*). (*E*) Photo of a patient beginning ambulation training with a right-sided below-knee amputation fitted with the X-Prosthesis and a contralateral F&F limb salvage technique with PMA/reverse sural flaps. (With Permission. Copyright 2020, Dr. Christopher Bibbo Main Street Enterprises, LLC, DBA Global Medicus.)

rings, preferably with skinny wires (**Fig. 12**B). The X-Prosthesis is placed onto the ExFix most commonly in the recovery room or on postoperative day 1. The length of X-Prosthesis length adjusted based on whether a low, standard length, or high amputation has been performed. Additional length and multiplanar angulation of the X-Prosthesis in relation to the residual limb is accommodated to maintain limb mechanical axis also is performed acutely, to allow smooth ambulation (see **Fig. 12**A). Half-pins are reliable when used in the tibia/femur cortex or when multiple rings are required for extremely large patients (**Fig. 12**C, D). Above-knee amputations require

ExFix construct to be built with half-pins on proximal femoral half or three-quarter rings (1 or 2 of these) and a distal femoral ring block (1 or 2). When knee contractures exist, a knee hinge on threaded rods that attaching the tibial and femoral rings facilitates gradual extension and protection of tendon lengthenings. The X-Prosthesis is designed to fit into standard ExFix ring holes, accepting 10-mm nuts. Rapid adjustable struts (Orthofix) are preferred as connectors, because these allow the surgeon and prosthetist to dial in the desired mechanical position and length of the limb. ST care is facilitated by windows in the cone, allowing in situ wound care and showering and providing drainage of fluid (see **Fig. 12**A, B). A quick-release mechanism allows for the X-Prosthesis to be detached easily from the ExFix for any reason, including wound inspection or any associated wound care needs. The X-Prosthesis can incorporate a hinged drop lock knee mechanism to allow knee motion during ambulation for above-knee amputations. The X-Prosthesis for immediate ambulation after hip disarticulation also is possible. Overall, the use of the X-Prosthesis has revolutionized patient rehabilitation and time to prosthetic fitting after major amputations of the lower extremity. The author has performed the X-Prosthesis on 1 limb and an F&F on the contralateral limb, allowing full, immediate weight bearing, entry into level 1 rehabilitation, early discharge to home, and accelerated placement of the permanent prosthesis (**Fig. 12**E). In summary, the X-Prosthesis is a novel IPOP that is easy to fit and mount and can be customized for the residual limb. The X-Prosthesis has improved the healing and rehabilitation after major lower extremity amputation surgery significantly and changed these patients' lives for the better.

DISCLOSURE

The author has nothing to disclose.

REFERENCES

1. Bibbo C. External fixator assisted immediate wound closure. Tech Foot Ankle Surg 2006;5:144–9.
2. Bibbo C. Foot and ankle surgery for chronic non-healing wounds. Surg Clin North Am 2020;100(4):707–25.
3. Bibbo C. Plantar heel reconstruction with a sensate plantar medial artery musculocutaneous pedicled island flap after wide excision of melanoma. J Foot Ankle Surg 2012;51(4):504–8.
4. Bibbo C, Stough J. Reduction calcaneoplasty and local muscle rotation flap as a salvage option for calcaneal osteomyelitis with soft tissue defect. J Foot Ankle Surg 2012;51(3):375–8.
5. Bibbo C. Reverse sural flap with bifocal Ilizarov technique for tibial osteomyelitis with bone & soft tissue defects. J Foot Ankle Surg 2014;53:344–9.
6. Bibbo C, Bauder A, Nelson J, et al. Reconstruction of traumatic tibia defects with free fibula flap and external fixation. Ann Plast Surg 2020. https://doi.org/10.1097/SAP.0000000000002240.
7. Bibbo C, Ehrlich DA, Kovach SJ. Pediatric lateral ankle physeal reconstruction by free microvascular transfer of the proximal fibular physis. J Foot Ankle Surg 2015;54(5):994–1000.
8. Bibbo C, Karnik SS, Albright JT. Ilizarov wound closure method for traumatic soft tissue defects. Foot Ankle Int 2010;31:628–33.
9. Bibbo C. A modification of the Syme amputation to prevent post-operative heel pad migration. J Foot Ankle Surg 2013;52:766–70.

10. Bibbo C, Ehrlich D, Levin LS, et al. Maintaining levels of lower extremity amputations. J Surg Orthop Adv 2016;25(3):137–48.
11. Bibbo C, Polga DJ, Mehta S, et al. General Principles of limb salvage versus amputation in Adults. In: Krajbich JI, Pinzur MS, Potter BK, et al, editors. Atlas of amputations and limb deficiencies. 4th edition. Chicago: America Academy of Orthopaedic Surgeons; 2016. p. 41–59. Chapter 4.

Surgical Treatment Protocol for Peripheral Nerve Dysfunction of the Lower Extremity: A Systematic Approach

Kaitlyn L. Ward, DPM[a],*, Edgardo R. Rodriguez-Collazo, DPM[b,c]

KEYWORDS

- Nerve pain • Peripheral nerve • Lower extremity • Nerve injuries • Neuroma
- Stump neuroma

KEY POINTS

- After an injury, if the process of nerve repair is incomplete or disrupted, a disorganized growth of neural tissue (neuroma) will result and may become painful.
- Common symptomatology of neuromas include sharp, burning, or electrical-like pain, most often at night, cold intolerance, paresthesias, and numbness.
- Nerve injuries were first classified by Seddon into 3 types: type I, neuropraxia; type II, axonotmesis; and type III, neurotmesis.
- Identification of nerve injury type should be performed with careful clinical examination, anesthetic blocks, and neurology assessment to obtain nerve conduction velocities and electromyography.

INTRODUCTION

Intractable nerve pain is a common and often debilitating complication after lower extremity trauma.[1] This often overlooked sequelae of injury stems from neuroma formation at the site of injury and can result in physical, psychological, social, and economic complications.[2–10] Effective, reproducible procedures to treat such injuries are necessary; however, owing to their complexity, there is no consensus on appropriate management.[6] Surgical intervention is often indicated for definitive treatment, requiring a thorough understanding of the degree and nature of the nerve injury.

[a] Complex Deformity Correction & Microsurgical Limb Reconstruction; [b] AMITA St. Joseph Hospital, St. Joseph Hospital-Manor Building, Attn: Podiatric Fellowship Office Room #425, 2913 Commonwealth Avenue, Chicago, IL 60657, USA; [c] Podiatric Medicine and Surgery Reconstructive Rearfoot/Ankle Surgery, Complex Deformity Correction & Microsurgical Limb Reconstruction
* Corresponding author. 730 Goodlette-Frank Road. #102, Naples, FL 34102.
E-mail address: Kaitlynlward@gmail.com

Clin Podiatr Med Surg 38 (2021) 73–82
https://doi.org/10.1016/j.cpm.2020.09.002
0891-8422/21/© 2020 Elsevier Inc. All rights reserved.
podiatric.theclinics.com

To conceptualize the appropriate management of any nerve pathology, it is imperative to understand the etiology of dysfunction. That is, when a nerve is traumatized, the proximal end will attempt to regenerate toward the distal segment in an effort to repair itself. If this process is incomplete or disrupted, a disorganized growth of neural tissue (a neuroma) will result, which may become painful.[4,6,8–10] Common symptomatology of neuromas include sharp, burning, or electrical-like pain, most often at night, cold intolerance, paresthesias, and numbness.[2–4,6,8–10]

Nerve injuries were first classified in 1943 by Seddon[11] into 3 types.[8] Neurapraxia (type I) is the least severe form of nerve injury. It typically occurs secondary to compressive trauma, resulting in a temporary block in conduction owing to local myelin damage. In such injuries, axons are not damaged and conduction studies will reveal normal amplitudes past the region of injury. Examples of compressive etiologies include localized injury or inflammation, mechanical irritation (tourniquet, cast, bandage, positioning, shoes, postural habits, repetitive ground reactive force), impinging anatomy (space occupying lesions), or true entrapment (scar tissue, fibrosis).

The second type, axonotmesis (type II) is more severe. It involves damage to the myelin and the axon, resulting in complete Wallerian degeneration of the distal nerve segment. Regeneration is possible in axonotmesis, because the epineurium and perineurium surrounding the nerve are preserved. In these injuries, internal degloving of the axon is present and amplitudes cannot normalize past the region of injury. As the proximal end of the nerve attempts to repair itself, the resulting aberrant nerve activity at the site of the injury results in neuroma formation, also known as a neuroma-in-continuity.[2,3] Common etiologies of such injuries include: traction injuries (sprains or fractures), direct trauma (significant contusions), or more severe or long-standing compressive etiologies previously mentioned.

Finally, the third form of nerve damage described by Seddon is neurotmesis (type III). This form is the most severe kind of nerve damage, which results in a total loss of physiologic function owing to complete disruption of the nerve (ie, iatrogenic neural transections or traumatic amputations).[1,4,6,9,10] As in a type II injury, the proximal or "live" end of the nerve continues to receive neural input and will often form a neuroma without an appropriate termination point or "grounding" of the nerve. Therefore, type III injuries represent end or "stump" neuromas.

More than 150 techniques for neuroma management have been described, which can make treatment of such injuries daunting.[10] As such, we describe our surgical treatment algorithm according to degree of injury as dictated by Seddon's classification based on the current literature for the treatment of lower extremity neurogenic pain.

METHODOLOGY

This protocol provides a framework to understand and surgically treat peripheral nerve injuries of the lower extremity. Basic principles and patient work-up are reviewed. Additionally, we highlight treatments based on the degree and nature of the nerve injury.

Obviously, patients necessitating surgical intervention should fail conservative efforts, including nonsteroidal anti-inflammatory drugs, topical anesthetics, physical therapy, and/or neuropathic pain medication.

Pertinent Electrophysiology and Diagnostic Studies

Before surgical intervention, a thorough, bilateral clinical and physical examination must be conducted. Typically, localized pain with percussion and generalized pain to the distribution of the affected nerve will be noted.[6] Preoperative local anesthetic blocks with corresponding pain relief should be used as a confirmatory test for nerve injury.[2–4,6] It is our recommendation to perform such blocks in the lower leg under ultrasound guidance, rather than the foot, to include all proximal nerve branches that may be affected. Patients must be counseled that the goal of surgery is pain relief and not improvement of sensation. In fact, postoperatively some degree of numbness should be expected.[6] Finally, evaluation by a neurologist is paramount to obtain bilateral nerve conduction velocities and electromyography (**Box 1** for an electromyogram/nerve conduction velocity interpretation reference guide).

Procedures

Fig. 1 is the algorithm we created and follow based on the available literature to date. Important considerations include the following.

- No paralytics are to be used during these cases. This should be discussed preoperatively with the anesthesiologist.

Box 1
Reference guide for nerve conduction velocity/electromyogram interpretation

Pneumonic: MLAA

- Myelin = latencies (ms)
- Latency: amount of stimulation needed for depolarization of the axons to elicit a response (spike)
  - Normal latencies: tibial and peroneal ~6 ms
- Axon = amplitudes (mV)
- Amplitude: amount of axons that can be depolarized
  - More axons intact = higher amplitude
  - Normal amplitudes
    - Tibial 4 mV
    - Peroneal 2 mV
- Conduction velocity = distance between stimulation sites/distance between latencies
  - Normal velocities
    - Approximately 40 m/s tibial and peroneal below knee
      - Less than 40 m/s abnormal
    - At least 10 m/s common peroneal nerve across the knee
- F wave = Diagnosis inflammatory neuropathies (Guillain-Barré syndrome)
- H reflex = To diagnose radiculopathies

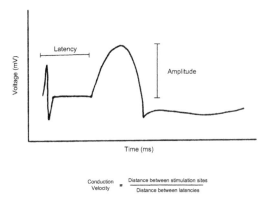

$$\text{Conduction Velocity} = \frac{\text{Distance between stimulation sites}}{\text{Distance between latencies}}$$

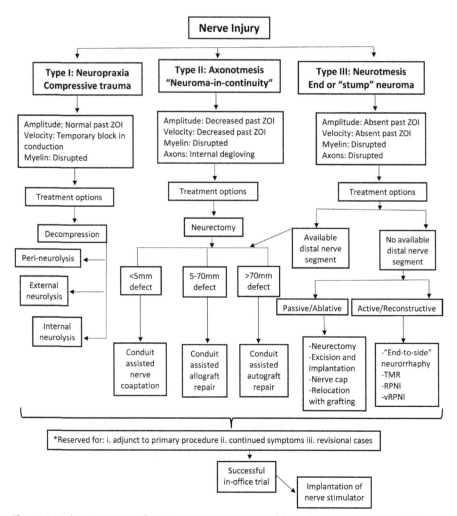

Fig. 1. Peripheral nerve dysfunction treatment protocol based on neuroma type. TMR, targeted muscle reinnervation; ZOI, zone of interest.

- We forgo the use of a tourniquet to prevent intraoperative compressive nerve trauma as well as to ensure meticulous dissection and hemostasis.
- Helpful intraoperative tools include the following items.
  - Nerve stimulator.
  - Loupe magnification and/or microscope (procedure dependent).
  - Micro instrument tray.
  - Local anesthetic with epinephrine, bipolar cautery, hydrogen peroxide, gel foam, and Surgicel for hemostasis.
  - Skin staples for atraumatic skin retraction at the beginning of the case and for final wound closure to allow the incision to drain and thus prevent hematoma formation.
- In all cases, the injured nerve must be repaired when it is on maximal stretch, so the foot and knee should be brought through full range of motion intraoperatively to ensure maintenance of the construct.

- We also use platelet therapy in these cases to promote angiogenesis, neovascularization, and pain reduction.[12]

Postoperative Care

After surgical intervention, we recommend admission for observation postoperatively. Patients should perform ankle and knee range of motion to prevent fibrosis at the surgical site. Physical therapy should evaluate the patient on postoperative day 1 to assist with partial weight bearing gait training. Elevation of the surgical limb above the level of the heart is paramount to prevent edema and subsequent neurogenic pain.

Our postoperative pain management consists of a patient-controlled analgesia pump, which is typically discontinued after 24 hours. After this, all narcotics are eliminated and a trimodal therapy approach, including gabapentin (Neurontin) (100 mg 3 times a day), tramadol (50 mg 3 times a day), and acetaminophen (Tylenol) (625 mg 3 times a day) is used. Patients are discharged when they are comfortable and can ambulate safely with the use of proper durable medical equipment. Upon discharge, tramadol and acetaminophen are continued for approximately 2 weeks. Gabapentin is typically continued for 3 months.

Patients are encouraged to weight bear as tolerated in a fracture boot upon staple removal (approximately 3–4 weeks postoperatively) and transition to normal shoe gear as tolerated at 4 to 6 weeks postoperatively.

DISCUSSION
Type I: Neuropraxia ("Compressive Trauma")

As mentioned elsewhere in this article, type I injuries typically result from compressive trauma. Consequently, treatment involves decompression and fasciotomy (**Fig. 2**), perineurolysis, external neurolysis, and/or internal neurolysis to allow the nerve to glide and function without inhibition.[2,3] These techniques also promote revascularization, regeneration, and nerve conduction by removing any mechanical obstructions.

Type II: Axonotmesis ("Neuroma-in-Continuity")

Type II nerve injuries represent neuromas-in-continuity (**Fig. 3**). In these cases, we recommend resecting the diseased segment of the nerve proximal to the zone of injury back to bleeding edges, which will result in a gap between the 2 nerve ends.[2,3,6,8] If the defect is less than 5 mm, conduit-assisted nerve coaptation should be performed. It is important to maintain a 2- to 3-mm gap between the 2 nerve ends within the conduit in

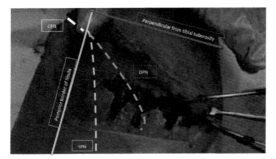

Fig. 2. Cadaveric representation of external fasciotomy over the lateral and anterior compartments. All inclusive of a standard decompression of the common peroneal nerve (CPN) and its associated branches. DPN, deep peroneal nerve.

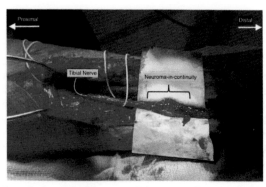

Fig. 3. Intraoperative photo of Seddon type II (neuroma-in-continuity) injury of the tibial nerve.

this technique (**Fig. 4**). If the resultant defect is between 5 and 70 mm, conduit-assisted allograft repair should be performed (**Fig. 5**). Again, it is important to keep an approximate 2- to 3-mm distance between the nerve and the allograft within the conduit. Finally, if the defect is greater than 70 mm, conduit-assisted autograft repair should be performed.

Type III: Neurotmesis (End or "Stump" Neuroma)

Type III nerve injuries include end or stump neuromas. In these instances, treatment depends on the availability of a distal nerve segment.[6] If the distal nerve segment is available, then the treatment protocol follows the same guidelines as type II nerve injuries. If the distal nerve segment cannot be found or the zone of injury will compromise the repair and coaptation, then passive and ablative or active and reconstructive procedures can be performed.[6]

Passive and ablative techniques include neurectomy, excision, and implantation (into bone, muscle, or vein), nerve cap, as well as nerve relocation with grafting.[1,6,9,10,13,14] Historically, these techniques have been commonly performed; however, the potential for recurrence of symptoms exists because they do not address the pathologic process of the proximal stump attempting to regenerate toward its distal target in an disorganized or incomplete fashion.[4,6,9,10] As with type II treatment recommendations, the goal of surgical intervention should be to give the axons of the proximal segment a termination point for any current aberrant nerve activity, thus giving the nerve a job to do in an organized manner to prevent recurrent neuroma formation.[2–4,6,9,10]

Owing to the shortcomings of passive procedures, a recent trend toward active/reconstructive procedures (end-to-side neurorrhaphy, targeted muscle reinnervation,

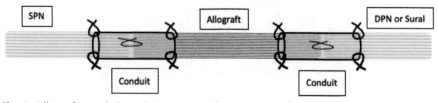

Fig. 4. Allograft-coupled conduit construct for nerve transfer. DPN, deep peroneal nerve; SPN, superficial peroneal nerve.

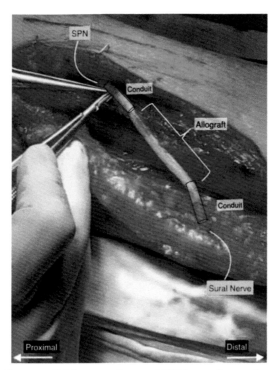

Fig. 5. Intraoperative superficial peroneal nerve (SPN) to sural nerve transfer (mid tibia).

regenerative peripheral nerve interfaces [RPNI], and vascularized RPNI [vRPNI]) have been reported.[4,6,9,10] It should be noted that these advanced techniques mandate microsurgical training for optimal results.

- End-to-side neurorrhaphy (also referred to as reverse end-to-side neurotization or end-to-side nerve repair): After neurectomy, the proximal stump is repaired to the side of an intact adjacent nerve by creating an epineural window or perineural disruption of the recipient nerve.[6]
- Targeted muscle reinnervation: After neurectomy, the proximal stump is repaired to a nearby muscular motor nerve branch (**Fig. 6**). This construct will serve to reinnervate the muscle from which the motor branch was harvested.[4]
- RPNI: After neurectomy, a free muscle cuff is wrapped around the proximal nerve stump. The aberrant axons work to innervate the muscular graft.[10]
- vRPNI: After neurectomy, a pedicled, vascularized muscle cuff is wrapped around the proximal nerve stump.[9] Again, the aberrant axons work to innervate the muscular graft.[10]

In end-to-side neurorrhaphy, targeted muscle reinnervation, RPNI, and vRPNI, the regenerating aberrant axons are provided a physiologic end-organ to satisfy the nerve endings to prevent or decrease symptomatic neuroma formation.[6] To date there are no studies comparing available active procedures, so it is our preference to select a procedure based on the available anatomy, bearing in mind the transfer needs to be performed in a well-cushioned, protected, traction-free environment. Furthermore, the possibility to combine active techniques exists (ie, neurorrhaphy with vRPNI) and

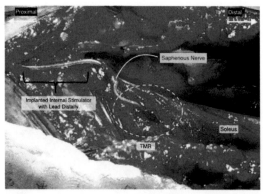

Fig. 6. Saphenous nerve to soleus muscle target muscle reimplantation (TMR).

preliminary results have been very promising in preventing painful neuroma formation, as well as phantom limb pain in amputees.[4,6,9,10] Currently, there are no studies directly comparing passive versus active repair; however, it is our preference to perform active procedures because they more appropriately address the underlying pathology.

Finally, recently the advent of implantable peripheral nerve stimulators has come to favor (**Fig. 7**). Because this neuromodulation system is relatively novel in the lower extremity, the literature is limited; however, our anecdotal evidence is promising. We first perform an in-office trial. If the trial is successful in providing some degree of pain relief, we move forward to inserting the device in the operating room (in an open fashion), to augment the primary procedure (ie, decompression, external neurolysis, and nerve transfer) or if there is continued pain in the revisional setting. Future studies are needed to appropriately evaluate the utilization of such devices and to provide clarity as to which patients are best suited for them.

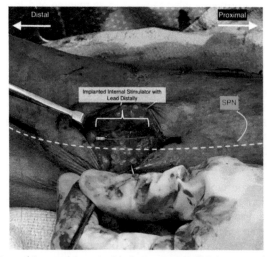

Fig. 7. Implantation of internal nerve stimulator at superficial peroneal nerve (SPN). Note that the lead is in close proximity to nerve; however, is not in direct contact.

SUMMARY

This protocol demonstrates the usefulness of a systematic algorithmic approach for treatment of peripheral nerve injuries. Currently, studies comparing techniques are lacking and will be necessary in the future to give more definitive treatment recommendations. It is our hope that by using this framework, along with scientific rationale and clinical judgment, the lower extremity surgeon can more readily incorporate this skillset into their armamentarium to address this complicated pathology.

CLINICS CARE POINTS

- Surgical treatment options are based on type of nerve injury.
- Type I (neuropraxia): Treatment for compressive injuries involve decompression, fasciotomy, perineurolysis, external neurolysis, and/or internal neurolysis to allow the nerve to glide and function without inhibition.
- Type II (axonotmesis): Treatment options depend on the gap size between the 2 nerve segments after resection of the neuroma-in-continuity.
  - Less than 5 mm = Conduit-assisted nerve coaptation
  - From 5 mm to 70 mm = Conduit-assisted allograft repair
  - Greater than 70 mm = Conduit-assisted autograft repair
- Type III (neurotmesis): Treatment options for end or stump neuromas depend on the availability of the distal nerve segment
  - If the distal nerve segment is available, the same protocol as type II injuries can be used.
  - If the distal nerve segment cannot be found or zone of injury is too compromised, passive and ablative or active and reconstructive procedures can be performed.
- Traditionally performed passive and ablative procedures do not address the pathologic process of neuroma formation. As such, a recent trend toward performing active and reconstructive procedures (end-to-side neurorrhaphy, targeted muscle reinnervation, RPNI, and vRPNI) has come into favor.
- Peripheral nerve stimulators can be used to augment a primary procedure or if there is continued pain in the revisional setting.

ACKNOWLEDGMENTS

The authors would like to thank Dr Roberto Segura. **Box 1** was synthesized on his findings from more than 30 years of experience.

DISCLOSURE

E. Rodriguez-Collazo is a consultant for Integra, Orthofix and Axogen. The authors declare that they have no relevant or material financial interests that relate to the research described in this article.

REFERENCES

1. Dellon A, Mackinnon S. Treatment of painful neuroma by neuroma resection and muscle implantation. J Plast Reconstr Surg 1986;77(3):427–38.
2. Bibbo C, Rodriguez-Collazo E. Nerve transfer with entubulated nerve allograft transfers to treat recalcitrant lower extremity neuromas. J Foot Ankle Surg 2017;56(1):82–6.

3. Bibbo C, Rodriguez-Collazo E, Finzen A. Superficial peroneal nerve to deep peroneal nerve transfer with allograft conduit for neuroma in continuity. J Foot Ankle Surg 2018;57(3):514–7.

4. Bowen JB, Wee CE, Kalik J, et al. Targeted muscle reinnervation to improve pain, prosthetic tolerance, and bioprosthetic outcomes in the amputee. Adv Wound Care (New Rochelle) 2017;6(8):261–7.

5. Ditty BJ, Omar NB, Rozzelle CJ. Chapter 24 - Surgery for Peripheral Nerve Trauma. In: Tubbs RS, Rizk E, Shoja MM, et al, editors. Nerves and Nerve Injuries. Amsterdam (Netherlands): Academic Press; 2015. p. 373–81. https://doi.org/10.1016/B978-0-12-802653-3.00073-7.

6. Eberlin K, Ducic I. Surgical algorithm for neuroma management: a changing treatment paradigm. Plast Reconstr Surg Glob Open 2018;6(10):e1952.

7. Public Affairs. "What is the U.S. Opioid Epidemic?" HHS.gov. 2019. Available at: https://Plus.google.com/+HHS; www.hhs.gov/opioids/about-the-epidemic/index.html.

8. Souza J, Purnell C, Cheesborough J, et al. Treatment of foot and ankle neuroma pain with processed nerve allografts. Foot Ankle Int 2016;37(10):1098–105.

9. Valerio I, Schulz SA, West J, et al. Targeted muscle reinnervation combined with a vascularized pedicled regenerative peripheral nerve interface. Plast Reconstr Surg Glob Open 2020;8(3):e2689.

10. Woo SL, Kung TA, Brown DL, et al. Regenerative peripheral nerve interfaces for the treatment of postamputation neuroma pain: a pilot study. Plast Reconstr Surg Glob Open 2016;4(12):e1038.

11. Seddon H. Three types of nerve injury. Brain 1943;66(4):237–88.

12. Gaiovych I, Savosko S, Labunets I, et al. Sciatic nerve regeneration after autografting and application of the bone marrow aspirate concentration. Georgian Med News 2019;(295):145–52.

13. Dellon A, Aszmann O. Treatment of superficial and deep peroneal neuromas by resection and translocation of the nerves into the anterolateral compartment. Foot Ankle Int 1998;19(5):300–3. https://doi.org/10.1177/107110798001900506.

14. Dellon A, Mackinnon S, Pestronk A. Implantation of sensory nerve into muscle: preliminary clinical and experimental observations on neuroma formation. Ann Plast Surg 1984;12:30–40.

Evaluation and Treatment of Foot Drop Using Nerve Transfer Techniques

Arshad A. Khan, DPM[a,b,]*,
Edgardo R. Rodriguez-Collazo, DPM[c,d,e], Erwin Lo, MD[f,g],
Asim Raja, DPM[h], Sujin Yu, MD[g], Hamid A. Khan, MD[g]

KEYWORDS

- Foot drop • Common peroneal nerve palsy • Radiculopathy • Nerve transfer
- Reinnervation

KEY POINTS

- Evaluation of foot drop begins by determining the etiologic cause. This is done by performing a thorough history and physical examination of the patient. Foot drop etiologic causes are then separated into three categories, the central nervous system, spinal nerve root injury, and distal peripheral nervous system foot drop.
- Diagnostic testing is an integral part when selecting procedure to be performed for foot drop correction. It is important to perform radiographic evaluation, EMG/NCV, ultrasound examination and MRI to rule help identify the origin of foot drop.
- Surgical considerations for foot drop are dependent upon the etiologic findings as well as diagnostic evaluation. Once identified these procedures can include the use of tendon transfers, nerve transfer procedures, and possible arthrodesis at the ankle joint.

 Video content accompanies this article at http://www.podiatric.theclinics.com.

---

[a] Department of Orthopedic Surgery, Indiana University School of Medicine, Gary/Northwest; [b] SpineTech, Brain and Spine Centers of Southeast Texas, 6025 Metropolitan Drive, Suite 205, Beaumont, TX 77706, USA; [c] Chicago Foot and Ankle Deformity Correction Center, 2913 North Commonwealth Avenue, Chicago, IL 60657, USA; [d] Reconstructive Foot & Ankle Fellowship Program, Saint Anthony Hospital; [e] Department of Pediatrics, Center for Excellence in Limb Lengthening and Reconstruction; [f] University of Texas Medical School, Mischer Neuroscience Institute, Houston, TX, USA; [g] SpineTech, Brain and Spine Center of Southeast Texas, 111 Vision Park Boulevard, Shenandoah, TX 77384, USA; [h] PMSR/RRA, Department of Orthopedics and Rehabilitation (DO&R), Womack Army Medical Center, 2817 Reilly Road, Fort Bragg, NC 28310, USA
* Corresponding author. SpineTech, Brain and Spine Centers of Southeast Texas, 6025 Metropolitan Drive, Suite 205, Beaumont, TX 77706.
E-mail address: aakdpm@gmail.com

Clin Podiatr Med Surg 38 (2021) 83–98
https://doi.org/10.1016/j.cpm.2020.09.004
0891-8422/21/© 2020 Elsevier Inc. All rights reserved.
podiatric.theclinics.com

INTRODUCTION

Foot drop, or drop foot, represents weakness to the tibialis anterior muscle, peroneal muscles, and extensor hallucis longus muscle. The condition is commonly attributed to traumatic or pathologic causes involving the central or peripheral nervous system. L4/L5 radiculopathy is recognized as the most common cause of drop foot. Injury to the common peroneal nerve (CPN) is recognized as the most frequently injured peripheral nerve of the lower extremity. Treatment outcomes are predominantly based on age, associated pathology, level of neural involvement, and duration of foot drop symptoms.

Muscular function secondary to motor loss can directly affect ankle joint motion and subtalar joint inversion. Patients commonly present with either complete or partial loss of function to the anterior and lateral muscle groups of the lower extremity. Heel strike and swing phase are commonly affected elements of the gait cycle. Heel strike is affected by decreased deceleration of plantarflexion (foot slap), whereas swing phase is affected by weakened, or absent, dorsiflexion at the ankle joint. This results in an inability of the digits to clear the ground. Compensation for these changes often leads to decreases in strength, balance, and the development of a steppage gait. Therefore, it is not uncommon for patients with drop foot to use various forms of braces and/or other assistive devices for stable ambulation.[1] Patients afflicted with foot drop symptoms can concomitantly suffer from neuropathic pain. Typical treatment of these individuals includes long-term neuropathic and narcotic medications.[1–6]

ETIOLOGY

Causes of foot drop are divided into two broad categories: conditions involving the central nervous system, and conditions involving the peripheral nervous system. The peripheral nervous system can further be subdivided into spinal nerve roots, distal peripheral nervous segments, and regions of the neuromuscular junction (NMJ). Establishing the true cause or origin of a drop foot condition is critical, because some lesions can mimic other lesions involving a different origin altogether. For example, such conditions as superior cluneal nerve entrapment neuropathy or CPN entrapment neuropathy can mimic lumbar-based pathology for drop foot.

The NMJ is where terminal axons meet muscle cell fibers. Pathologic conditions affecting the NMJ can involve presynaptic membranes, the synaptic cleft, or postsynaptic membranes. Altered NMJ function can adversely affect the ability for muscle cells to depolarize and contract. Because of this complexity, treatment options for such conditions require multidisciplinary consultation for initiating appropriate treatment and rehabilitation.

Central Nervous System Drop Foot Etiologies

Causes for drop foot involving the central nervous system include

- Upper motor neuron, medial motor cortex fiber compression, as they descend to the ventral gray matter of the spinal cord
- Microvascular lacunar syndromes of the brain associated with intracapsular and cerebral peduncle
- Masses or tumors
- Stroke affecting the anterior cerebral artery of the interhemispheric motor cortex in the homunculus
- Myelopathy of the spinal cord extrapyramidal tract
- Charcot-Marie-Tooth disease

- Multiple sclerosis
- Cerebral palsy
- Muscular dystrophy
- Polio
- Amyotrophic lateral sclerosis

Spinal Nerve Root Foot Drop Etiology

- Lumbar L4/L5
  - Compression/inflammation
    - Nerve root
    - Herniated nucleus pulposus
    - Foraminal stenosis
    - Bone spurs
    - Facet cysts
    - Ligamentum flavum
    - Tumors and masses
    - Pregnancy
    - Iatrogenic

Distal Peripheral Nervous System Foot Drop Etiology

- Peripheral nerve entrapment[7–21]
- Inflammatory neuropathy
- Direct trauma to the nerve
- Bone tumors of proximal fibula
- Ganglion cyst
- Intraneural tumors
- Vascular pathology
- Leprosy
- Compression at the level of the proximal fibular head

Kadiyala and colleagues[22] performed cadaveric evaluations on 19 limbs, finding fewer intraneural blood vessels to the CPN (at the level of the fibular neck), as opposed to an abundant vascular supply from the tibial artery supplying the posterior tibial nerve (**Fig. 1**).

SURGICAL TREATMENT OPTIONS

Current treatment options for foot drop lack randomized control trials. Most surgical treatment options cited in the literature involve small case studies. Treatment of spine nerve root–related foot drop at the level of L5 includes lumbar discectomy or decompression of the nerve root, or roots. Patients responding well to lumbar surgery had a shorter duration of foot drop, were generally younger, and had better preoperative strength rating of the tibialis anterior muscle.

Treatment options available for distal peripheral nervous system foot drop include decompression and neurolysis, nerve grafting, nerve transfer, and tendon transfers.

Surgical neurolysis of the CPN is indicated in patients who have not responded to conservative management. Causes of neurolysis include functional impairment of the nerve, nerve pain, and abscess. Terzis and Kostas[23] had good to excellent results in 62 patients who underwent microneurolysis and nerve decompression, or a reconstructive nerve procedure. Kim and colleagues[24] found 88% improvement following neurolysis in their study of peroneal nerve lesions at the level of the knee.

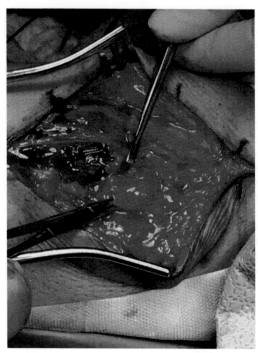

Fig. 1. Intraoperative picture of ganglion cyst surrounding the common peroneal nerve.

Nerve grafting for treating lesions of the peroneal nerves have been described in the literature. Kim and Kline[25] performed intrafascicular nerve grafting on patients associated with peroneal nerve lesions of greater than 3 cm. Their study noted the use of shorter graft lengths leading to more successful outcomes.

Nerve transfers have been described to treat injuries of the hip and knee. Nerves used for transfer include either a branch of the tibial or superficial peroneal nerve into the deep peroneal, or into a motor branch of the tibialis anterior muscle. Nath and colleagues[26] reported on 21 patients having 80% improvement of dorsiflexion and eversion after performing nerve transfers.

Tendon transfers are considered for foot drop when the primary muscle group is unresponsive to direct muscle stimulation, or unable to respond to an electrical stimulus. The second caveat when considering this option is for the existence of surrounding muscle groups to function normally with stimulation. Tendon transfer procedures include transferring the posterior tibial tendon into the cuneiforms of the midfoot, and stabilizing the construct with anchors or interference screws (**Fig. 2**). The bridal procedure is a modification of posterior tibial tendon transfer, by anastomosing the posterior tibial tendon to the peroneus longus and the anterior tibial tendons. Cho and colleagues[27] reported on patients having undergone anterior transfers of the posterior tibial tendon with satisfactory functional outcomes and the ability to regain 33% of ankle dorsiflexion as compared with the contralateral/unaffected ankle.[2,22,24–49]

PREOPERATIVE CLINICAL EVALUATION

Preoperative clinical assessment begins with a thorough evaluation of the patient's history and review of systems. Surgical history is integral to determining cause of

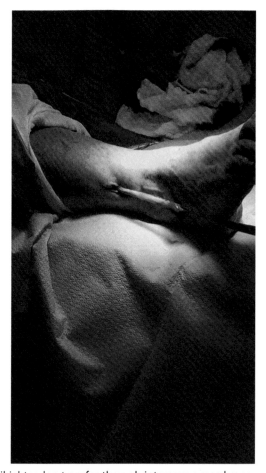

Fig. 2. Posterior tibial tendon transfer through interosseus membrane.

foot drop. Important factors also include the patient's age, duration of symptoms, and comorbidities. Previous diagnostic studies need to be identified (radiographs, MRIs, or electromyography/nerve conduction velocity of the lower extremities), because they are important for comparative analysis before formulating a treatment plan.

Physical Examination

A thorough physical examination needs to include information regarding the central and peripheral nervous system. Thus, evaluating the lower back to rule out any lumbar spine related cause is recommended via multidisciplinary consultation.

When evaluating the lower extremities, it is important to identify any bony abnormalities or deformities. The authors have identified several patients with compression of the CPN secondary to ankle joint–related injuries. On examination, proximal palpation of both fibular heads may reveal a notable prominence associated with the injured side. Proximal fibular head/neck subluxation can equate to pathologic traction on the CPN, with subsequent symptoms noted distally (**Fig. 3**).

Nitz and colleagues[46] reported on 66 patients demonstrating electrophysiologic deficits to the CPN following grade 2 or grade 3 ankle sprains. Brassell and

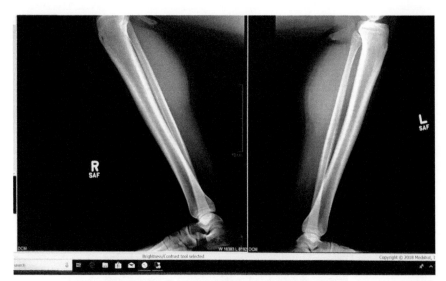

Fig. 3. Weightbearing lateral tibia and fibula views of bilateral lower extremities with the knee in 20° of flexion at the knee joint. The right fibula bone is noted to be anteriorly displaced when compared to the contralateral film following and ankle sprain.

colleagues[47] likewise reported on the evaluation and treatment of CPN injuries following ankle sprains.

Muscle strength evaluation should be performed from the proximal upper leg down to the foot. Bilateral evaluations are performed to highlight any differences or discrepancies between the two extremities. Examination should include assessments for muscle atrophy, strength/weakness, and motor/sensory deficits. Patients are also asked to perform the rapid foot tap test by placing the evaluator's hand under each foot and having the patients tap the evaluator's hand as quickly as possible.

Diagnostic Transcutaneous Electrical Nerve Stimulation Testing

Diagnostic muscle testing is performed by direct muscle stimulation using transcutaneous electrical nerve stimulation (**Fig. 4**). This is done primarily to differentiate between conditions in which conduction signals from motor nerves are not reaching an otherwise normal target muscle group, or that the muscle itself is incapable of responding to any uninhibited conduction signal meant to innervate the muscle group complex.

The tibialis anterior, peroneal brevis, and peroneal longus are commonly tested muscles in most drop foot cases. A grounding pad is placed on the vastus medialis muscle just proximal to the knee. Acupuncture needles are used for direct stimulation and placed within the corresponding muscles being tested. Placement of the needles should begin along the proximal aspect of the muscle and gradually moved distal as needed. This allows for accurate assessments of the type of motion being identified and recorded (**Fig. 5**). Muscle groups demonstrating absent or diminished contractions from direct needle stimulation may be indicative of pathology to the muscle itself. This means conduction signaling to the muscle may be normal and uninterrupted, but the muscle fibers are unable to elicit a response to the stimulation received.

However, if dorsiflexion is observed with direct muscle stimulation, then the muscle unit is functional and the problem may exist with the inability of electrical signals to

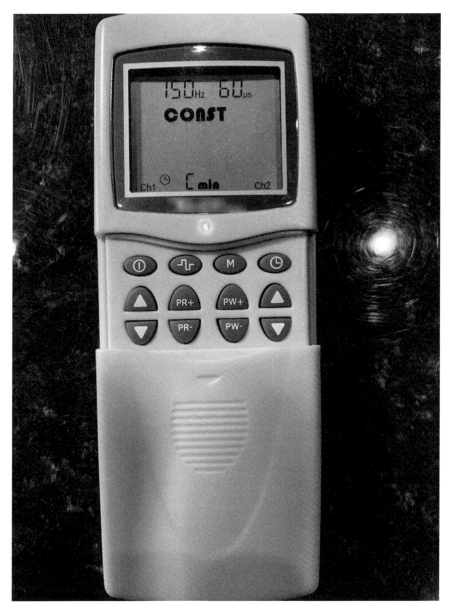

Fig. 4. Transcutaneous electrical nerve stimulation used for direct muscle stimulation.

reach the muscle group complex. With further investigation (for all conditions caused by motor nerve impingement, entrapment, or injury) such patients may be considered for nerve decompression, or nerve transfer type procedures.

Diagnostic Nerve Block

The authors perform a diagnostic nerve block of the CPN behind the fibula at the level of the tibial tuberosity and fibular neck. The block is generally performed on patients with causes of weakness in dorsiflexion emanating from the spinal nerve root. Tajiri

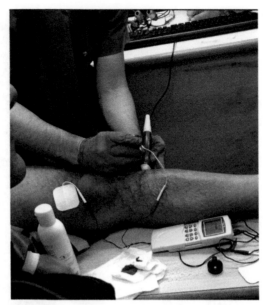

Fig. 5. Placement of grounding pads to Vastas Medialis muscle and placement of stimulating needle with ultrasonography to Tibialis Anterior muscle.

and colleagues[48] reported on the use of CPN blocks to effectively block pain to the lower extremity from associated disk herniation. Sangwan and colleagues[49] also reported similar findings in their study.

Our diagnostic nerve block consists of 3 mL of lidocaine plain, which is infiltrated directly behind the proximal fibular head/neck region. Although the CPN is in the area of lidocaine infiltration, the injection does not specifically target the CPN. Intuitively, with administration of a local anesthetic around the CPN one would expect to see further weakening, or exacerbation, of drop foot symptoms. However, in most patients with etiologic causes originating from a spinal nerve root injury, a paradoxic effect tends to occur. Individuals experience a reversal of their foot drop symptoms, with concomitant decreases in lower back pain, and increased sensation to distal regions of neuropathy. The diagnostic nerve block is transient and lasts anywhere from a few hours to a few days, after which the patient's symptoms normally return. The paradoxic nature of the injection in this patient population is currently under institutional review board–directed clinical investigation. Our current general consensus is that it is not based on hydrodissection of soft tissues around the CPN. Barret describes what he has termed, the "Phoenix sign," in which an increase in muscle strength of the foot extensors is observed, following administration of local anesthetic around the common peroneal nerve.[50–69] Likewise, similar postdiagnostic injection increases in dorsiflexion with partial to complete resolution of foot drop symptoms have also been observed in a clinical setting by the authors (**Fig. 6**).

Diagnostic Testing

Electromyography/nerve conduction velocity
Patients are referred for electromyography and nerve conduction studies before surgical intervention. Such diagnostic modalities help differentiate nerve root issues of the spine from neuropathic and/or myopathic lesions of the peripheral nerves. Certain

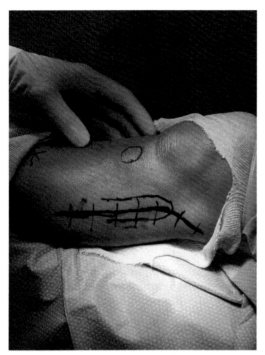

Fig. 6. *Circle* represents the tibial tuberosity and the fibula is *outlined*. An 8 to 10 cm curvi-linear incision placed over the proximal fibula.

compression neuropathies expressed and/or exacerbated by dynamic loads may not always be identifiable using electromyography/nerve conduction velocity type modalities. In such situations, testing for repetitive plantarflexion has been advocated as a more reliable means for identifying these specific types of entrapment neuropathies.

MRI/magnetic resonance neurography
MRI is used for evaluation of the lower back and for peripheral nerves when ruling out tumors or compression/impingement type conditions. Conventional MRI imaging for proximal peripheral nerves may be difficult to assess, in which case magnetic resonance neurography may provide a better option for purposes of assessment. Magnetic resonance neurography works by directly imaging nerves and identifying nerve root entrapments within the spine, not always detected by conventional spinal MRI.

Ultrasound evaluation
Ultrasound is useful to rule out abscesses, masses, trauma, and tumors. Tsukamoto and colleagues[62] reported on identifying axonal damage to the CPN by using ultrasound examination to evaluate its cross-sectional area. Ultrasound is also a valuable tool for peripheral nerve block placement, with avoidance of accidental intraneural or intravascular infiltration/placement.

Radiographic evaluation
Plain film imaging is commonly used to rule out fractures, joint subluxation/dislocations, or bony abnormalities. When considering injury or traction to the CPN, the proximal fibula should be evaluated by obtaining bilateral knee films for comparison. The lateral view should be performed at 20° of knee flexion while standing. This is to

identify any anterior or lateral displacement of the proximal fibula. The authors have identified fibular subluxation as a consequence of previous ankle trauma, or as a consequence of repetitive ankle inversion injuries.

Procedure selection

For lesions directly involving the CPN or its branches, surgical decompression with additional external neurolysis is advocated for release of compression and/or entrapment. Intraoperative use of nerve stimulators (Checkpoint Stimulator/Locator, Checkpoint Surgical, Cleveland, OH), either before or following decompression/external neurolysis, is advocated for intraoperative assessments of returned function following nerve stimulation. If function returns (ie, dorsiflexion) following decompressive measures, then nothing further is warranted. If dorsiflexion at the ankle cannot be elicited with stimulation following comprehensive decompression, then sequential stimulation along the course of the deep peroneal nerve is conducted until dorsiflexion is elicited. A nerve transfer is then planned to the exact same location at which a positive ankle joint response (ie, dorsiflexion) was elicited. Nerves selected for transfer/grafting are commonly taken from either a motor branch of the tibial or superficial peroneal nerve.

If the patient has foot drop associated with a more proximal spinal root nerve lesion, a targeted muscle reinnervation using a muscular branch of the tibial nerve from the gastrocnemius muscle is considered for transfer to the CPN. We believe this works because the tibial nerve originates within the lumbosacral plexus (anterior division), with nerve root levels of L2, L3, L4, L5, S1, S2, and S3. The CPN originates from the posterior division with nerve root levels of L2, L3, L4, L5, S1, and S2. It is the S3 component of the tibial nerve that we theorize bypasses the CPN spinal nerve root lesion, allowing motor impulses to reach musculature of the lower leg.

PROCEDURAL APPROACH
Patient Positioning

Patient is placed in the supine position with attention directed to the patient's proximal tibia. This region is used for acquisition of blood for concentrating bone marrow aspirate (Magellan Autologous Concentration System, Isto Biologics, Hopkinton, MA). A small incision is made to place an aspiration needle into the proximal tibia. A Luer lock syringe is used to evacuate 60 mL of bone marrow aspirate from the tibia, which is processed for generating concentrated bone marrow aspirate. A nurse or anesthesiologist may additionally remove 30 mL of peripheral whole blood from the patient for the acquisition of platelet-rich plasma.

The leg is then placed on a sterile, well-padded, surgical triangle to prevent excessive pressure in the region of the popliteal fossa. The leg is slightly internally rotated at the hip by using a blanket roll (see **Fig. 3**).

Incision Placement

The patient's lower leg is now marked by outlining the tibial tuberosity and the fibular head. An arrow is drawn from the tibial tuberosity to the proximal fibula. Next the skin is marked with a curvilinear incision that is approximately 8 to 10 cm in length and slightly posterior to the fibula (**Fig. 7**).

Dissection Technique

Using loupe magnification, the incision is carefully deepened through the skin and soft tissue using sharp and blunt dissection and bipolar cauterization. It should be noted that the neural and vascular structures reside deep to the fascia at this level, so it is

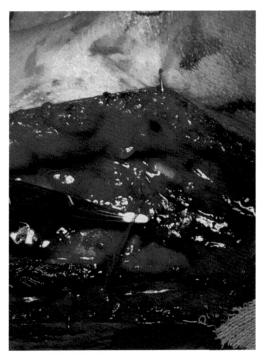

Fig. 7. End-to-side suturing of muscular branch from the tibial nerve transferred to the common peroneal nerve.

imperative that care be taken when incising the fascia over the compartments of the lower extremity. The authors use a malleable retractor to help protect the neural and vascular structures beneath the fascia, as it is incised using a tenotomy scissor. The CPN is found near the proximal aspect of the fascial release. In some patients the CPN is adherent to the overlying fascia, and may inadvertently experience iatrogenic injury based on being mistaken for underlying adipose tissue.

Identification and Stimulation of the Common Peroneal Nerve

On reflection of the deep fascia, the proximal fibula and the posterior compartment of the leg are identified. Intraoperative functional examination of the CPN is performed by using a nerve stimulator (Checkpoint Stimulator/Locator, Checkpoint Surgical). Motor defects to the nerve are observed with stimulation testing (Video 1). In some situations of impingement, or injury at the level of the CPN, weakness associated with dorsiflexion and protonation might be observed. Similarly, with lesions more proximal at the level of the lumbar spine, there can still be weakness noted with nerve stimulation of the CPN specifically.

Decompression of the Posterior Compartment

Attention is then directed to the posterior compartment, where the deep fascia is incised between the gastrocnemius and soleus muscle bellies. The demarcation between the two muscles is identified and the interface between the gastrocnemius and soleus is carefully opened and any residual fascia over either muscle is removed.

Identification of Tibial Motor Branch

An intraoperative nerve stimulator is now used at its lowest setting (generally 0.5 mA), and swept slowly across the gastrocnemius muscle belly. Evidence of a visible contracture of a segment of the gastrocnemius aids in identifying the location of an intramuscular motor branch with which to perform the nerve transfer. Once a muscular branch is identified, it is dissected out further proximally and distally for acquisition of length. Planning for adequate nerve length facilitates a transfer without tension. When performing the necessary nerve transposition from the posterior to the lateral compartment, a vessel loop is placed near the motor nerve harvest site and rotated to the region of the CPN. Once adequate length has been verified, the tibial nerve motor branch can safely be transected at its NMJ and subsequently transposed and sutured to the CPN with an end-to-side nerve anastomosis.

End-to-Side Nerve Anastomosis

A window is created in the epineurium of the CPN, proximal to the bifurcation of the deep peroneal and superficial peroneal nerves, or distal to the region of entrapment (if the lesion involves the CPN itself). Motor nerve anastomosis is performed under microscope assistance with 8–0 nylon or Prolene suture. Once suturing is complete, stimulation of the motor branch is performed using a nerve stimulator to assess contractibility of the tibialis anterior muscle. Additional motor branch anastomosis is conducted to the CPN, using the same end-to-side technique. This is done if intraoperative testing does not elicit a strong enough response to the target muscle.

On completion, the nerve anastomosis interface is sprayed with bone marrow aspirate concentrate along with platelets and calcium chloride. The nerve transfer site can further be protected with a nerve conduit, or amniotic membrane of choice. The fascia is not reapproximated because of possible postoperative nerve compression and scarring.

Skin closure is performed using 2–0 Vicryl and 3–0 Monocryl in a subcuticular fashion and Derma-bond with pernio is applied. Dressings consist of Kerlix, ABD, and a large Ace bandage wrapped above the knee to help prevent excessive flexion at the knee joint.

RECOVERY AND REHABILITATION

Postoperative dressings are not removed for approximately 7 to 10 days. Patients are able to ambulate immediately in a closed toe shoe as tolerated. The two main restrictions include: avoiding excessive flexion at the knee joint and not removing the postoperative dressings.

Patients should be counseled preoperatively with regards to increased edema of the operative extremity. Edema management involves the use of compression socks after the incision site has healed. Once the incision site is healed, the patient is then referred for physical therapy for proprioceptive muscle training and continued electrical stimulation.

SUMMARY

When considering surgical management for the treatment of drop foot, it is first and foremost imperative to establish the cause of the condition. Keep in mind that not all etiologies resulting in clinical drop foot have surgical options. Second, establishing a cause allows the provider to more appropriately curtail a multidisciplinary approach to work-up and ultimately treat the patient. Lastly, understanding of the cause allows for a more appropriate selection of surgical treatment options available to the patient. To date, the authors have performed more than 30 successful procedures and have been able to restore function, proprioceptive stability, and muscle strength. Many of our targeted nerve transfer patients relate a significant improvement to their quality of life, with activities of daily living and recreational activities previously hindered by weakness and/or pain. Postoperatively, we have seen patient activity levels increase with discontinuation of ambulatory assist devices, and a discontinuation of the need to use braces. Several of our patients have experienced associated weight loss with the increase in activity levels. We have also noted a decrease in pain levels in our patients with direct correlation to decrease in neuropathic pain medications and narcotic use in our patients.

CLINICS CARE POINTS

- Identification of the cause of foot drop is imperative to formulate an effective treatment plan.
- Evaluation by a spine surgeon and neurologist must be carried out before any treatment is performed for foot drop.
- If the cause of foot drop is not from direct trauma to the CPN or its branches, then a complete decompression of the CPN may be unnecessary.
- Patients that have direct traumatic injury to the pelvis and the nerve root in this area do not respond well to targeted muscle reinnervation for foot drop and may be a candidate for a tendon transfer.

DISCLOSURE

No funding was received and there are no conflicts of interest for any authors.

SUPPLEMENTARY DATA

Supplementary data related to this article can be found online at https://doi.org/10.1016/j.cpm.2020.09.004.

REFERENCES

1. Wiszomirska I, Błażkiewicz M, Kaczmarczyk K, et al. Effect of drop foot on spatio-temporal, kinematic, and kinetic parameters during gait. Appl Bionics Biomech 2017;2017:3595461.
2. Liu K, Zhu W, Shi J, et al. Foot drop caused by lumbar degenerative disease: clinical features, prognostic factors of surgical outcome and clinical stage. PLoS One 2013;8(11):e80375.
3. Krych AJ, Giuseffi SA, Kuzma SA, et al. Is peroneal nerve injury associated with worse function after knee dislocation? Clin Orthop Relat Res 2014;472:2630–6.
4. Huckhagel T, Nüchtern J, Regelsberger J, et al. Nerve trauma of the lower extremity: evaluation of 60,422 leg injured patients from the TraumaRegister DGU between 2002 and 2015. Scand J Trauma Resusc Emerg Med 2018;26(01):40.
5. Aprile I, Caliandro P, La Torre G. Multicenter study of peroneal mononeuropathy: clinical, neurophysiologic, and quality of life assessment. J Peripher Nerv Syst 2005;10(03):259–68.
6. Carolus AE, Becker M, Cuny J, et al. The Interdisciplinary management of foot drop. Dtsch Arztebl Int 2019;116(20):347–54.
7. Westhout FD, Paré LS, Linskey ME. Central causes of foot drop: rare and underappreciated differential diagnoses. J Spinal Cord Med 2007;30(1):62–6.

8. Goetz CG. Textbook of clinical neurology. Philadelphia (PA): WB Saunders; 2003.
9. Marich EN. Human anatomy and physiology. 6th edition. San Francisco (PA): Pearson Benjamin Cummings; 2004.
10. Blumenfeld H. Neuroanatomy through clinical cases. Sunderland (MA): Sinauer Associates Inc; 2002.
11. Yamauchi T, Kim K, Isu T, et al. Undiagnosed peripheral nerve disease in patients with failed lumbar disc surgery. Asian Spine J 2018;12(4):720–5.
12. Kim JY, Kim DK, Yoon SH. Isolated painless foot drop due to cerebral infarction mimicking lumbar radiculopathy: a case report. Korean J Spine 2015;12(3): 210–2. https://doi.org/10.14245/kjs.2015.12.3.210.
13. Stewart JD. Foot drop: where, why and what to do? Pract Neurol 2008;8:158–69.
14. Frontera WR, Silver JK. Essentials of physical medicine and rehabilitation. St. Louis (MO): Mosby; 2002.
15. Gilchrist RV, Bhagia SM, Lenrow DA, et al. Painless foot drop: an atypical etiology of a common presentation. Pain Physician 2002;5:419.
16. Ma J, He Y, Wang A, et al. Risk factors analysis for foot drop associated with lumbar disc herniation: an analysis of 236 patients. World Neurosurg 2018;110: e1017–24.
17. Samson D, Ng CY, Power D. An evidence-based algorithm for the management of common peroneal nerve injury associated with traumatic knee dislocation. EFORT Open Rev 2017;1(10):362–7.
18. Suntrup-Krueger S, Schilling M, Schwindt W, et al. Case report of bilateral relapsing-remitting sciatic nerve palsy during two pregnancies. BMC Res Notes 2015;8:654.
19. Han Y, Kim KT, Cho DC, et al. Misunderstanding of foot drop in a patient with Charcot-Marie-Tooth disease and lumbar disk herniation. J Korean Neurosurg Soc 2015;57(4):295–7.
20. Lisovski V, Minderis M. Intraneural ganglion cyst: a case report and a review of the literature. Acta Med Litu 2019;26(2):147–51.
21. Nikolopoulos D, Safos G, Sergides N, et al. Deep peroneal nerve palsy caused by an extraneural ganglion cyst: a rare case. Case Rep Orthop 2015;2015:861697.
22. Kadiyala RK, Ramirez A, Taylor AE, et al. The blood supply of the common peroneal nerve in the popliteal fossa. J Bone Joint Surg Br 2005;87(3):337–42.
23. Terzis JK, Kostas I. Outcome with microsurgery of common peroneal nerve lesions. J Plast Reconstr Aesthet Surg 2020;73(1):72–80.
24. Kim DH, Murovic JA, Teil RL, et al. Management and outcomes in 318 operative common peroneal nerve lesions at the Louisiana State University Health Sciences Center. Neurosurg 2004;54(6):1421–9.
25. Kim DH, Kline DG. Management and results of peroneal nerve lesions. Neurosurgery 1996;39(2):312–9, discussion 319–320.
26. Nath RK, Lyons AB, Paizi M. Successful management of foot drop by nerve transfers to the deep peroneal nerve. J Reconstr Microsurg 2008;24(6):419–27.
27. Cho BK, Park KJ, Choi SM, et al. Functional outcomes following anterior transfer of the tibialis posterior tendon for foot drop secondary to peroneal nerve palsy. Foot Ankle Int 2017;8:627–33.
28. Jeon S, Kim DY, Shim DJ, et al. Common peroneal neuropathy with anterior tibial artery occlusion: a case report. Ann Rehabil Med 2017;41(4):715–9.
29. Choe W. Leprosy presenting as unilateral foot drop in an immigrant boy. Postgrad Med J 1994;70(820):111–2.
30. Bhargava D, Sinha P, Odak S, et al. Surgical outcome for foot drop in lumbar degenerative disease. Glob Spine J 2012;2(3):125–8.

31. Takenaka S, Aono H. Prediction of postoperative clinical recovery of drop foot attributable to lumbar degenerative diseases, via a Bayesian network. Clin Orthop Relat Res 2017;475(3):872–80.

32. Fiume D, Sherkat S, Callovini GM, et al. Treatment of the failed back surgery syndrome due to lumbo-sacral epidural fibrosis. Acta Neurochir Suppl 1995;64:116–8.

33. Rohde V, Mielke D, Ryang Y, et al. The immediately failed lumbar disc surgery: incidence, aetiologies, imaging and management. Neurosurg Rev 2015;38:191–5.

34. Jakubowitz E, Jao D, Windhagen H, et al. Treatment options for neurogenic foot drop: a systematic literature research. Z Orthop Unfall 2017;155:402–8.

35. Terzis JK, Kostas I. Outcomes with microsurgery of common peroneal nerve lesions. J Plast Reconstr Aesthet Surg 2020;73(1):72–80.

36. Morimoto D, Isu T, Kim K, et al. Microsurgical decompression for peroneal nerve entrapment neuropathy. Neurol Med Chir (Tokyo) 2015;55:669–73.

37. Richard B. Surgical management of neuritis. Kathmandu, Nepal: Ekta Books; 2004.

38. Nath RK, Somasundaram C. Gait improvements after peroneal or tibial nerve transfer in patients with foot drop: a retrospective study. Eplasty 2017;17:e31.

39. Giuffre JL, Bishop AT, Spinner RJ, et al. Partial tibial nerve transfer to the tibialis anterior motor branch to treat peroneal nerve injury after knee trauma. Clin Orthop Relat Res 2012;470(3):779–90.

40. Bodily KD, Spinner RJ, Bishop AT. Restoration of motor function of the deep fibular (peroneal) nerve by direct nerve transfer of branches from the tibial nerve: an anatomical study. Clin Anat 2004;17(3):201–5.

41. Flores LP, Martins RS, Siqueira MG. Clinical results of transferring a motor branch of the tibial nerve to the deep peroneal nerve for treatment of foot drop. Neurosurgery 2013;73(4):609–15, discussion 615-606.

42. Johnson JE, Paxton ES, Lippe J, et al. Outcomes of the bridle procedure for the treatment of foot drop. Foot Ankle Int 2015;36(11):1287–96.

43. Krishnamurthy S, Ibrahim M. Tendon transfers in foot drop. Indian J Plast Surg 2019;52(1):100–8.

44. Ho B, Khan Z, Switaj PJ, et al. Treatment of peroneal nerve injuries with simultaneous tendon transfer and nerve exploration. J Orthop Surg Res 2014;9:67.

45. Alastair Compston, Aids to the investigation of peripheral nerve injuries. Medical Research Council: nerve injuries Research Committee. His Majesty's Stationery Office: 1942; pp. 48 (iii) and 74 figures and 7 diagrams; with aids to the Examination of the Peripheral Nervous System. By Michael O'Brien for the Guarantors of Brain. Saunders Elsevier: 2010; pp. [8] 64 and 94 Figures, Brain, Volume 133, Issue 10, October 2010, Pages 2838–2844, https://doi.org/10.1093/brain/awq270.

46. Nitz AJ, Dobner JJ, Kersey D. Nerve injury and grades II and III ankle sprains. Am J Sports Med 1985;13(3):177–82.

47. Brassell J, Marder B, Miller J. Key considerations with ankle sprains and common peroneal nerve traction injuries. Podiatry Today 2019;32(9).

48. Tajiri K, Takahashi K, Ikeda K, et al. Common peroneal nerve block for sciatica. Clin Orthop Relat Res 1998;(347):203–7.

49. Sangwan SS, Mittal R, Kundu ZS, et al. Prolapsed intervertebral disc with sciatica: the role of common peroneal nerve block. Trop Doct 2005;35(3):172–4.

50. Barrett S. How the "phoenix sign" can predict the success of nerve decompression. Podiatry Today 2018;31(5).

51. Tehrani KHN. A study of nerve conduction velocity in diabetic patients and its relationship with tendon reflexes (T-reflex). Open Access Maced J Med Sci 2018;6(6):1072–6.

52. Won YH, Kim KW, Choi JT, et al. Correlation between muscle electrophysiology and strength after fibular nerve injury. Neurol Sci 2016;37:1293–8.

53. Kwon HK, Kim L, Park YK. Compound nerve action potential of common peroneal nerve and sural nerve action potential in common peroneal neuropathy. J Korean Med Sci 2008;23(1):117–21.

54. Chhabra A. Incremental value of magnetic resonance neurography of lumbosacral plexus over non-contributory lumbar spine magnetic resonance imaging in radiculopathy: a prospective study. World J Radiol 2016;8(1):109.

55. Dong Q, Jacobson JA, Jamadar DA, et al. Entrapment neuropathies in the upper and lower limbs: anatomy and MRI features. Radiol Res Pract 2012;2012:230679.

56. Iwamoto N, Kim K, Isu T, et al. Repetitive plantar flexion test as an adjunct tool for the diagnosis of common peroneal nerve entrapment neuropathy. World Neurosurg 2016;86:484–9.

57. Charles JA, Souayah N. EMG/NCS in the evaluation of spine trauma with radicular symptoms. Neurol Clin Pract 2013;3(1):8–14.

58. Van den Bergh FR, Vanhoenacker FM, De Smet E, et al. Peroneal nerve: normal anatomy and pathologic findings on routine MRI of the knee. Insights Imaging 2013;4(3):287–99.

59. Chen Y, Haacke EM, Li J. Peripheral nerve magnetic resonance imaging. F1000Res 2019;8:F1000. Faculty Rev-1803.

60. Muniz Neto FJ, Kihara Filho EN, Miranda FC, et al. Demystifying MR neurography of the lumbosacral plexus: from protocols to pathologies. Biomed Res Int 2018; 2018:9608947.

61. Kim K, Isu T, Kokubo R, et al. Repetitive plantar flexion (provocation) test for the diagnosis of intermittent claudication due to peroneal nerve entrapment neuropathy: case report. NMC Case Rep J 2015;2:140–2.

62. Tsukamoto H, Granata G, Coraci D, et al. Ultrasound and neurophysiological correlation in common fibular nerve conduction block at fibular head. Clin Neurophysiol 2014;125:1491–5.

63. Almeida Silvares PR, Fernandes Guerreiro JP, Müller SS, et al. Acute isolated anterolateral dislocation of the proximal tibiofibular joint. Rev Bras Ortop 2015;45(4): 460–4.

64. Milankov M, Kecojević V, Gvozdenović N, et al. Dislocation of the proximal tibiofibular joint. Med Pregl 2013;66(9–10):387–91.

65. Hey HW, Ng LW, Ng YH, et al. Radiographical definition of the proximal tibiofibular joint - A cross-sectional study of 2984 knees and literature review. Injury 2016;47(6):1276–81.

66. Rodriguez-Collazo E, Tamire Y. J Open surgical implantation of viable cryopreserved placental membrane after decompression and neurolysis of the common peroneal nerve: a case series. Orthop Surg Res 2017;12(1):88.

67. Bacci ED, Coyne KS, Poon JL, et al. Understanding side effects of therapy for myasthenia gravis and their impact on daily life. BMC Neurol 2019;19(1):335.

68. Reife MD, Coulis CM. Peroneal neuropathy misdiagnosed as L5 radiculopathy: a case report. Chiropr Man Therap 2013;21(1):12.

69. Chan CW, Peng P. Failed back surgery syndrome. Pain Med 2011;12:577–606.

Membrane-Induced Technique for the Management of Combined Soft Tissue and Osseous Defects

Ryan Pereira, DPM[a], William C. Perry, DPM[b],
Peter A. Crisologo, DPM[c], Michael D. Liette, DPM[d],
Bryan Hall, DPM[c], Shawkat Ghazal Hafez Hassn, MD[e],
Suhail Masadeh, DPM[f],*

KEYWORDS

- Bone defect • Induced membrane • Masquelet technique

KEY POINTS

- The induced membrane technique is a simple, effective, and reproducible 2-staged procedure for the management of segmental bone defects.
- The first stage consists of aggressive debridement to remove all nonviable tissue and placement of a polymethylmethacrylate spacer.
- The cement spacer induces a foreign body reaction, leading to the formation of a vascularized bioactive membrane, and secretes growth factors, which promote bone regeneration.
- The second stage consists of careful dissection and preservation of the formed membrane, followed by the placement of autogenous bone graft to fill the osseous defect.
- The induced membrane technique is limited by the amount of autogenous bone graft required to fill the deficit. It is associated with increased morbidity at the autograft harvest site.

[a] Private Practice, Anastasia Medical Group, 1301 Plantation Island Drive S, Suite 203A, Saint Augustine, FL 32080, USA; [b] University of Cincinnati Medical Center, Cincinnati Veteran Affairs Medical Center, Veterans Affairs Hospital, 3200 Vine Street, Cincinnati, OH 45220, USA; [c] Department of Surgery, Division of Podiatric Surgery, University of Cincinnati Medical Center, 231 Albert Sabin Way, ML 0513, Cincinnati, OH 45276, USA; [d] Division of Podiatric Surgery, University of Cincinnati Medical Center, 231 Albert Sabin Way, ML 0513, Cincinnati, OH 45276, USA; [e] General Organization of Teaching Hospitals and Neuromuscular Institute, 1 Altayar Fekry Street, Embaba, Gizza, Cairo 11865, Egypt; [f] Division of Podiatric Surgery, University of Cincinnati Medical Center, Cincinnati. Veteran Affairs Medical Center, 231 Albert Sabin Way, ML 0513, Cincinnati, OH 45276, USA
* Corresponding author.
E-mail address: masadesb@uc.edu

Clin Podiatr Med Surg 38 (2021) 99–110
https://doi.org/10.1016/j.cpm.2020.09.005
0891-8422/21/Published by Elsevier Inc.
podiatric.theclinics.com

INTRODUCTION

The management of segmental bone defects of the lower extremity remains a difficult challenge. Bone loss can occur secondary to trauma or after surgical debridement of necrotic, infected, or neoplastic bone.[1] Reconstructive techniques are determined by the size and length of the osseous defects. Although autogenous bone grafting remains the gold standard for small bone defects, larger bone defects can be managed with acute shortening, distraction osteogenesis, or a vascularized free bone transfer.[2,3] Despite the success of these techniques, they have their inherent complications and remain technically challenging. Furthermore, these techniques often require the prolonged use of external fixators, which is often associated with poor patient tolerance. Masquelet[4,5] described a 2-stage technique for the management of posttraumatic infected nonunions. This technique provides a simple and reproducible method to manage bone loss independent of defect size and length. The surgeon must understand the meticulous nature of the technique to achieve success (**Fig. 1**).

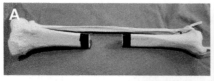 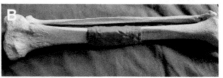

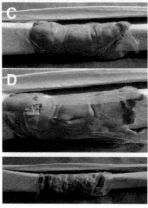

Fig. 1. (*A*) Induced membrane technique summary. The first step in stage I is an aggressive and deliberate debridement of all nonviable tissue. The proximal and distal segments are decorticated approximately 2 cm as represented by the black tape; the medullary canal is debrided especially after the removal of infected intrameduallry fixation. Multiple tissue samples are obtained for microbiological and histologic examination. (*B*) Second step in stage I is the placement of a PMMA cement spacer. The cement spacer is fashioned and placed in the deficit to include medullary placement as well as 2 cm surrounding the distal ends of the bone. The spacer should be large enough to provide stability and maintain tension on the soft tissue without compromising closure. The segments can be stabilized with and external fixator or a K-wire inserted within the spacer. (*C*) Step 1 in stage II. At 6 to 8 weeks, the space is explanted. Care must be taken to preserve the membrane while removing the spacer. Osteotomes may be used to remove the cement in pieces without disturbing the membrane. The medullary canal and bone ends are debrided, and multiple tissue samples obtained again for microbiology. (*D*) Step 2 of stage II. The deficit and medullary canal are tightly packed with autogenous cancellous bone graft or from a reamer irrigator aspirator system. If the deficit is too large, Allograft (osteoinductive and osteoconductive) may be added to the autogenous graft to increase bulk.

TECHNIQUE

The concept of the induced membrane technique is based on the physiologic reaction that occurs in the presence of an implanted foreign body.[6] This reaction leads to the formation of a bioactive membrane that secretes growth factors critical in the bone healing process.[6,7]

The induced membrane technique involves a 2-stage process. During the first stage, a radical debridement of all nonviable tissue is performed until healthy bleeding margins are achieved. This critical step is often underappreciated in the management of these difficult cases. The goal is to create a biological environment free of necrotic or infected tissue by complete excision of all nonviable osseous and soft tissue structures. Inadequate debridement negatively effects the quality of the formed membrane and increases the risk of a recurrent infection.[2,8,9] The removal of sclerotic bone achieved when adequate bone bleeding is obtained ensures the viability of the remaining bone and is recognized clinically by the presence of punctate bleeding within the medullary canal, otherwise known as the "paprika sign."[9]

Once adequate debridement is achieved, a polymethylmethacrylate (PMMA) cement block is embedded within the defect. The cement block should extend approximately 1 cm into the medullary canal and circumferentially over the cortices to cover the exposed bone ends by approximately 2 cm, similar to the morphology

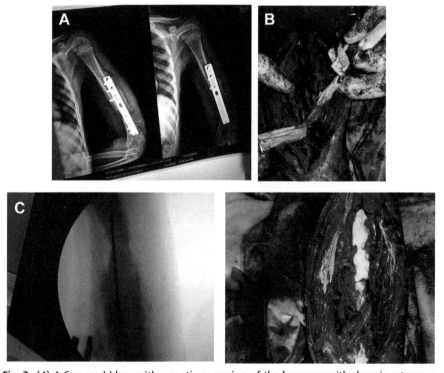

Fig. 2. (*A*) A 6-year-old boy with a septic nonunion of the humerus with chronic osteomyelitis and discharging sinus with retained hardware. He underwent extensive debridement with a resultant 10-cm bone deficit. (*B*) Postdebridement 10-cm gap. (*C*) Placement of PMMA spacer with intramedullary wire for stability. Clinical photograph of spacer in situ. ([*A*] *Courtesy of* S. G. H. Hassn, MD, Cairo, Egypt.)

of a joint capsule. The intramedullary and extramedullary placement improves stability and encourages the formation of a continuous membrane from both ends of the bone defect. The spacer should be larger than the original defect without compromising the soft tissues.[6] During polymerization, the spacer should be removed or surrounded with a wet sponge to avoid heat necrosis to the surrounding tissue from the exothermic reaction that occurs as the spacer hardens.[2] Additional stability of the spacer can be achieved with a wire or an external fixator to avoid micromotion. Micromotion can lead to the formation of a fragile and poorly vascularized membrane, which can affect osseous consolidation. If a soft tissue defect is present, a local, regional, or free flap is performed during the first stage procedure. The cement spacer is left in place for 6 to 8 weeks to allow for the development and maturation of the induced membrane[2,6,7,9] (**Figs. 2** and **3**).

During the second surgical stage, the membrane is identified and carefully incised to provide access to the spacer with a longitudinal incision made beyond the margin of the defect to avoid disruption of the membrane's delicate vascularity. The cement spacer is removed in pieces with the use of osteotomes to avoid membrane compromise. The ends of the bones are decorticated, and the medullary canal is debrided of any remaining cement. This process creates an open medullary channel on both ends of the exposed bone. Tissue samples are obtained from multiple sites and sent for microbiological analysis. Cancellous autograft is then harvested and implanted within

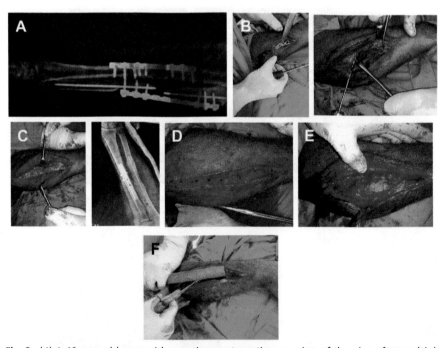

Fig. 3. (*A*) A 40-year-old man with aseptic symptomatic nonunion of the ulna after multiple operations with persistent nonunion for 6 years. (*B*) Removal of hardware and debridement of all nonviable tissue. (*C*) Placement of cement spacer for a 10-cm deficit s/p debridement. (*D*) Primary closure of the wound. (*E*) Removal of the spacer at 6 weeks. Note the formation of the bioactive membrane. (*F*) A 10-cm gap between bone ends. (*G*) Placement of autogenous corticocancellous graft with fixation and preservation of the membrane. Internal fixation of defect. ([*A*] *Courtesy of* S. G. H. Hassn, MD, Cairo, Egypt.)

G

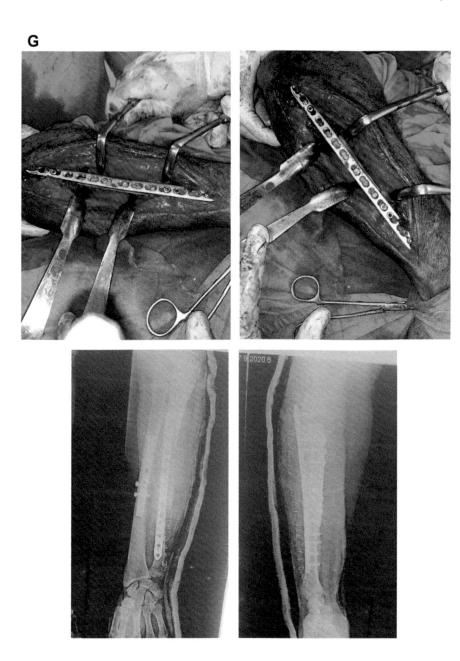

Fig. 3. (*continued*).

the membrane to fill the defect. The bone graft must be packed tightly, and the membrane approximated with suture over the graft. If there is evidence of infection during the second stage, the first stage must be repeated by excising the membrane and debriding the defect. During the second stage, definitive fixation is used to stabilize the bone segments.[6] Rigid fixation promotes vascularization of the graft while flexible fixation enhances corticalization[6] (see **Fig. 3**; **Fig. 4**).

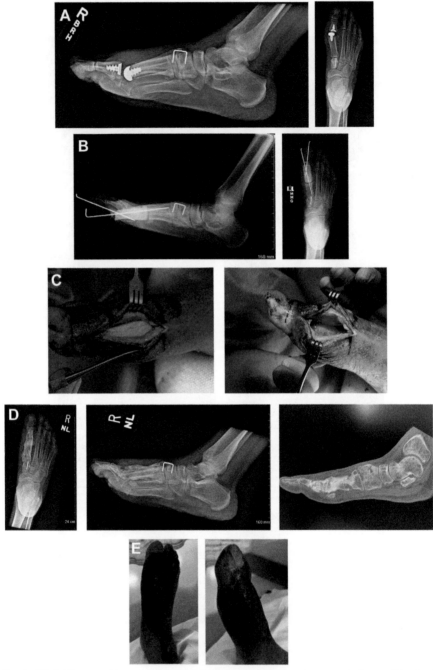

Fig. 4. (*A*) A 60-year–old man with a failed septic total first metatarsal phalangeal implant. (*B*) Explant of the total joint, debridement, and placement of an antibiotic spacer fixated with K-wires. (*C*) Upon removal of the cement spacer, a 4.8-cm deficit is noted. Note the induced membrane after removal of the antibiotic spacer. (*D*) Consolidation of the cancellous bone graft after 6 months and a 4.8-cm deficit, the construct was stabilized with an external fixator during the healing process. A computed tomography scan demonstrates consolidation. (*E*) Clinical picture showing complete healing in good position and alignment. ([*A*] *Courtesy of* B. Hall, DPM, Cincinnati, OH.)

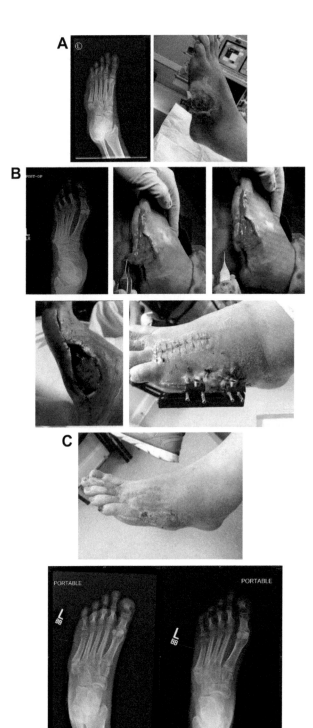

DISCUSSION

The decision to proceed with limb salvage in cases of bone defects remains challenging and is based on multiple local and systemic factors. The location and size of the bone defect, vascular and neurologic status of the limb, as well as the age and comorbidities of the patient are key components of the decision-making process.[1,5,10] Masquelet and colleagues[2,4,5] described their induced membrane technique for the management of large segmental bone defects of 25 cm or less. This technique is most frequently reported in the management of defects of long bones, with the tibia as the most common site described. However, several investigators have reported on the success of this technique at other anatomic sites.[3] The benefits of the induced membrane technique include the prevention of fibrous and soft tissue interposition, maintenance of soft tissue tension, and enhancement of graft vascularization while simultaneously avoiding graft resorption.[2,11,12]

The body's response to a PMMA spacer leads to the formation of a highly vascularized pseudosynovial membrane.[13] A histologic and biochemical evaluation of the membrane in a rabbit model at multiple time points during the formation of the induced membrane has been described previously.[13] This analysis was able to identify and describe the structure, function, and time course of growth factor production during membrane formation and maturation. The initial phase of membrane formation is characterized by an inflammatory reaction present with multinucleated giant cells and localized edema. At 2 weeks, the external surface of the membrane is composed of capillaries, fibroblasts, myofibroblasts, and collagen, whereas the fibrous inner membrane exhibits a synovial-like epithelium. The inflammatory reaction and edema are decreased at 4 weeks. Capillaries penetrate the entire membrane and the outer membrane capillaries increase in size. After 6 to 8 weeks, the edema resolves, and few inflammatory cells remain. Biochemical analysis demonstrated a high concentration of growth factors, specifically vascular endothelial growth factor and transforming growth factor beta-1. The concentration of vascular endothelial growth factor and transforming growth factor beta-1 remain high throughout the formation and maturation of the induced membrane. Conversely, the concentration of bone morphogenic protein 2 is time dependent, with the greatest concentration present between 4 and 8 weeks of membrane development.[2] These growth factors play a key role in graft vascularization and bone formation.[14,15] Performing the second stage at the appropriate time of peak growth factor concentration is largely responsible for the success of this technique.

Giannoudis and colleagues[16] published a series of 43 patients, including 3 metatarsal cases, with a defect size of between 2 and 5 cm. They reported a 93% union

---

Fig. 5. (A) A 43-year-old woman with uncontrolled diabetes and an infected nonunion of the fifth metatarsal (right). Patient with a soft tissue abscess to the lateral foot (left). (B) Placement of antibiotic spacer. Use of the induced membrane technique in a small defect and a compromised host. The wound was debrided including bone and soft tissue, and antibiotic spacer was placed in the 1-cm deficit and local flap coverage with an abductor digit minimi muscle flap and split thickness skin graft with stabilization via and external fixator. Muscle inset. Skin graft placement. Placement of external minifixator. (C) At 6 weeks, the flap was elevated, the spacer was removed, and the induced membrane with filled with autogenous cancellous bone graft from the calcaneus. Clinical picture of the healed flap and consolidated fracture site. Radiographic appearance of the consolidated fracture. ([A, Right] Courtesy of R. Pereira, DPM, Saint Augustine, FL.)

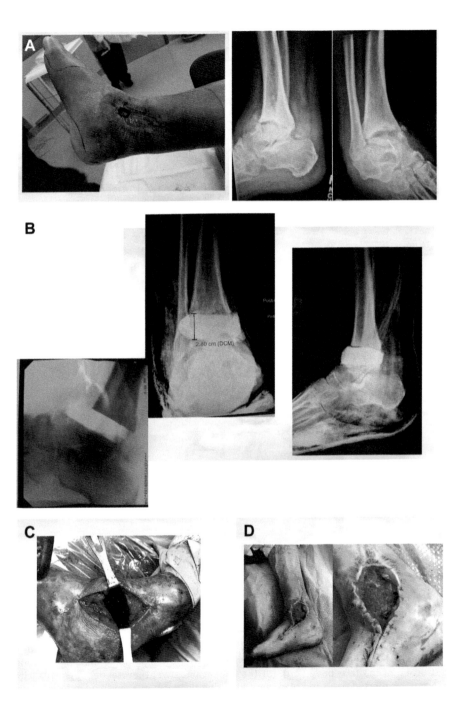

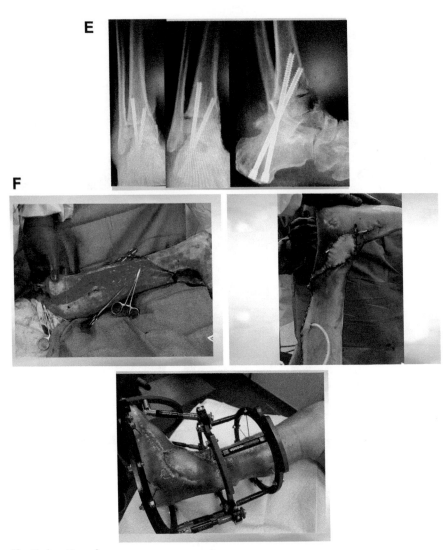

Fig. 6. (*continued*).

Fig. 6. (*A*) A 50-year-old patient with previous history of medial malleolus fracture presented with a draining sinus septic ankle joint (*right*). Radiographic imaging showing destruction of the talar body (*left*). (*B*) The patient underwent several debridements with resection of infected bone and placement of antibiotic spacer in a modified induced membrane technique. The deficit size is approximately 2.8 cm. (*C*) Removal of the spacer. (*D*) Placement of a corticocancellous graft and allograft (iliac crest + autogenous bone + bone marrow aspirate + femoral head allograft). (*E*) Internal fixation of the graft and deficit. (*F*) Coverage of the soft tissue defect with a reverse sural artery flap and application of external fixation. Flap inset and flap healing. ([*A, Right*] *Courtesy of* S. Masadeh, DPM, Cincinnati, OH.)

rate with an average time to healing of 1.24 months per centimeter of defect.[16] There are several other studies published that use the induced membrane technique with good clinical and radiographic outcomes. However, high-level evidence-based studies are lacking.[2] Future studies to address optimal fixation, type of cement, anatomic sites, timing of the second stage procedure, and the use of this technique in various comorbidities such as diabetes is needed.[3] Existing data are favorable to consider the induced membrane technique as a viable option for the treatment of patients with significant bone loss (**Figs. 5** and **6**).

SUMMARY

Management of bone loss secondary to trauma, infection, or oncologic resection remains challenging. Various techniques have been described to reconstruct these deficits. The induced membrane technique provides a simple and reproducible technique for the management of bone loss. Although high-quality prospective studies are needed, the current literature is encouraging. A multidisciplinary approach must be used when the decision for reconstruction is made to determine the ideal treatment method, especially in cases with combined soft tissue and bone loss.

CLINICS CARE POINTS

- The induced membrane technique is a 2-stage process for the management of osseous defect with a 6- to 8-week optimal time between stages.
- Aggressive and deliberate debridement is a crucial step for a successful outcome.
- Tissue samples for microbiological testing is critical for the evaluation of infection control.
- The cement spacer provides a mechanical and biological role by preventing fibrous interposition between bone segments and inducing the formation of a vascular membrane that secrets growth factors.
- The induced membrane technique requires autologous cancellous graft that is inserted into the formed membrane.

DISCLOSURE

The authors have nothing to disclose.

REFERENCES

1. Mauffrey C, Barlow BT, Smith W. Management of segmental bone defects. J Am Acad Orthop Surg 2015;23(3):143–53.
2. Taylor BC, French BG, Fowler TT, et al. Induced membrane technique for reconstruction to manage bone loss. J Am Acad Orthop Surg 2012;20(3):142–50.
3. Masquelet A, Kanakaris NK, Obert L, et al. Bone repair using the Masquelet technique. J Bone Joint Surg Am 2019;101(11):1024–36.
4. Masquelet A, Fitoussi F, Begue T, et al. Reconstruction of the long bones by the induced membrane and spongy autograft. Ann Chir Plast Esthet 2000;45(3):346-53.
5. Masquelet AC. Muscle reconstruction in reconstructive surgery: soft tissue repair and long bone reconstruction. Langenbecks Arch Surg 2003;388(5):344–6.
6. Masquelet AC. Induced membrane technique: pearls and pitfalls. J Orthop Trauma 2017;31(Suppl 5):S36–8.

7. Gruber HE, Ode G, Hoelscher G, et al. Osteogenic, stem cell and molecular characterisation of the human induced membrane from extremity bone defects. Bone Joint Res 2016;5(4):106–15.

8. Aurégan J-C, Bégué T. Induced membrane for treatment of critical sized bone defect: a review of experimental and clinical experiences. Int orthopaedics 2014;38(9):1971–8.

9. Chadayammuri V, Hake M, Mauffrey C. Innovative strategies for the management of long bone infection: a review of the Masquelet technique. Patient Saf Surg 2015;9:32.

10. DeCoster TA, Gehlert RJ, Mikola EA, et al. Management of posttraumatic segmental bone defects. J Am Acad Orthop Surg 2004;12:10.

11. Pelissier P, Martin D, Baudet J, et al. Behaviour of cancellous bone graft placed in induced membranes. Br J Plast Surg 2002;55(7):596–8.

12. Viateau V, Bensidhoum M, Guillemin G, et al. Use of the induced membrane technique for bone tissue engineering purposes: animal studies. Orthop Clin North Am 2010;41(1):49–56 [table of contents].

13. Pelissier PH, Masquelet AC, Bareille R, et al. Induced membranes secrete growth factors including vascular and osteoinductive factors and could stimulate bone regeneration. J Orthop Res 2004;22(1):73–9.

14. Pfeilschifter J, Diel I, Scheppach B, et al. Concentration of transforming growth factor beta in human bone tissue: relationship to age, menopause, bone turnover, and bone volume. J Bone Miner Res 1998;13(4):16.

15. Riley EH, Lane JM, Urist MR, et al. Bone morphogenetic protein-2: biology and applications. Clin Orthop Relat Res 1996;324:39–46.

16. Giannoudis PV, Harwood PJ, Tosounidis T, et al. Restoration of long bone defects treated with the induced membrane technique: protocol and outcomes. Injury 2016;47:S53–61.

Management of Osseous Defects in the Tibia

Utilization of External Fixation, Distraction Osteogenesis, and Bone Transport

Kelsey Millonig, DPM, MPH[a],*, Byron Hutchinson, DPM[b]

KEYWORDS

- Segmental bone defects • Distraction osteogenesis • Corticotomy • Regenerate
- Bone transport

KEY POINTS

- Distraction osteogenesis provides solutions for segmental defects, lessening the need for grafts, enabling dynamization, adaptability for adjustments, and providing an option for large defects.
- Corticotomy techniques are numerous and consideration for techniques is important for preventing thermal necrosis. Optimal placement is near metaphyseal bone for vascularity.
- Understanding the latency period, distraction, and regenerate phases is critical.
- There are anatomic soft tissue considerations with wire placement, gradual lengthening for neurovascular adaptation, and implications on regenerate.

The use of external fixators has revolutionized treatment options for segmental bone defects in the tibia. Distraction osteogenesis and bone transport are techniques that offer utility for osseous defects once considered unmanageable.[1,2] Several external fixation constructs can be employed, including monolateral or circular fixation. The authors prefer using an orthogonal circular external fixator for tibial segmental defects. Although these techniques continue to evolve over time, there are several key considerations.

INDICATIONS

Segmental defects often develop in the tibia from explantation of hardware, including total ankle replacements, trauma including malunion or nonunions, osteomyelitis,

[a] Rubin Institute of Advanced Orthopedics, International Center for Limb Lengthening, 2401 W Belvedere Avenue, Baltimore, MD 21215, USA; [b] CHI Franciscan Advanced Foot and Ankle Fellowship, Franciscan Foot and Ankle Associates, 16233 Sylvester Road Southwest, Burien, WA 98166, USA
* Corresponding author.
E-mail address: Kelsey.J.Millonig@gmail.com

Clin Podiatr Med Surg 38 (2021) 111–116
https://doi.org/10.1016/j.cpm.2020.09.006
0891-8422/21/© 2020 Elsevier Inc. All rights reserved.

podiatric.theclinics.com

avascular necrosis, and neoplasms. The use of distraction osteogenesis or bone transport offers many advantages:

1. Eliminating the necessity for large autografts that have poor results with axial loading and allowing adequate marginal resection without concern for defect size[3]
2. Enabling dynamization that promotes bone healing through axial loading
3. Frame adjustments support loading the bone segment for regenerate consolidation and the ability to change positioning, length, and biomechanical environment
4. Corticotomy enhances vascularity[4]

Distraction osteogenesis, also known as external limb lengthening, is the more ideal treatment choice for segmental tibial defects 5 cm or less (**Fig. 1**). Although more complex, bone transport or internal limb lengthening offers a unique solution to larger segmental defects greater than 5 cm in length and is a utility for a poor soft tissue envelope when an incision may not be possible (**Fig. 2**). However, in the authors' experience, the drawbacks of bone transport include a high learning curve and the challenges posed by docking site healing.

CORTICOTOMY TECHNIQUES

The first essential piece to successful distraction osteogenesis is the corticotomy. There are several key factors to consider for the corticotomy including the prevention of thermal osteonecrosis to enhance regenerate.[1,5–8] The location of the corticotomy is important, as metaphyseal bone has the best vascularity with larger surface area and therefore has higher healing potential. Numerous corticotomy techniques exist.

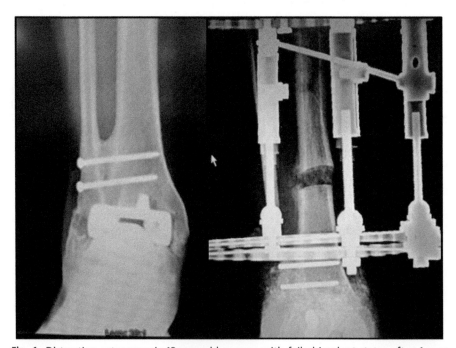

Fig. 1. Distraction osteogenesis 43-year-old woman with failed implant status after 4-year total ankle replacement. Patient underwent primary tibiocalcaneal fusion with distal tibial lengthening.

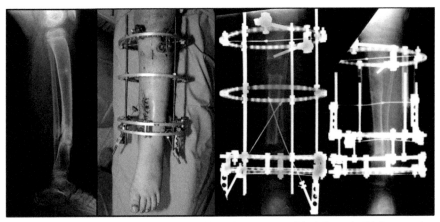

Fig. 2. Internal bone transport 12-year-old male trauma with infected tibial nonunion. (*Courtesy of* M. Samchukov, MD, Dallas, TX.)

Classic

This is an open incision technique. Osteotomize the medial and lateral cortex. The remaining corticotomy is completed with rotational osteoclasis utilizing circular rings.

Multiple Drill Holes

This uses small anterior incisions. A 4 to 5 mm diameter drill is used to create a series of drill holes around the anterior two-thirds of the bone circumference; an osteotome is used to connect the drill holes to complete the osteotomy, and the posterior cortex is broken.

Gigli Saw

Percutaneous incisions are made with subperiosteal tunnels created with critical necessity to clear soft tissue from the undersurface of the saw. The gigli saw is tied to suture and passed from 1 transverse incision to the other and pulled through the bone[9,10]

Focal Dome

This is a semicircular-shaped osteotomy with the center of rotation of angulation (CORA) corresponding to the center of the circular cut and the point of rotation for the dome. This is primarily used for acute correction of angular deformities in conjunction with lengthening and is the authors' preferred technique when angulation is present and not direct lengthening.

Power Saw

This technique requires greater disruption of blood flow secondary to greater exposure necessary and higher potential for thermal osteonecrosis. However, the technique offers enhanced simplicity and greater ability for acute wedge correction with angulation.

Minimally Invasive Systems

New minimally invasive osteotomy systems are available that allow osteotomy to be completed via 3 to 5 mm incisions with continuous irrigation.

LATENCY

The latency phase allows the local biologic environment to initiate a healing response to the corticotomy and is critical prior to distraction. The standard latency period is considered 3 to 10 days.[11–14] However, additional factors that impede bone healing may necessitate longer latency, such as comorbidities, immunosuppressive therapy, or infection. One of the authors (B.H.) has significant experience with revision surgery and prefers a latency period of 7 to 14 days.

DISTRACTION

The most widely accepted distraction rate is 1 mm per day completed in 0.25 mm increments, 4 times daily. However, increasing rhythm can yield improved bone formation and may be necessary in areas where healing may be compromised secondary to soft tissue injury or recurrent trauma.[5] Patient compliance is also of concern with distraction. The authors have found that a distraction rate of 0.5 mm to 0.7 mm per day is more suitable for segmental defects of the tibia.

REGENERATE

Adequate regenerate formation depends on mechanical and biologic conditions; therefore metabolic optimization of the patient preoperatively including vitamin D levels and thyroid levels should be evaluated. Bone regenerate requires bone remodeling and eventual consolidation. The process of regeneration evolves from mechanical stress of gradual stretching of the soft tissues in the bone segment gaps, yielding a cascade of cellular events to produce intramembranous bone formation and callotasis.[1,5,6,11] The process of consolidation can be supplemented through controlled axial loading and dynamization. Tricortical radiographic consolidation on 2 orthogonal radiographs is the most common definition for consolidation used as an indicator for removal of the external fixation.[15] In addition, intraoperative radiographic stress of the regenerate can be completed to determine stability, which the author employs. Two numeric parameters assist in evaluation of regenerate:

1. Distraction-consolidation time (DCT): consolidation time is often twice as long as distraction time in children and 3 to 4 times as long in adults.
2. Healing index (HI): measured as DCT/cm is 1 mo/cm in children and 2 to 3 mo/cm in adults.[15]

However, because of the wide clinical indications for distraction osteogenesis bony consolidation should be assessed on a patient-to-patient basis.

SOFT TISSUE

With distraction, soft tissues will be stretched and experience trauma with wire placement. Joint range of motion and muscle distraction are proportionally affected with the lengthening employed. The soft tissue can affect regenerate formation also; for example, strong muscle groups such as the posterior group in the lower extremity can yield procurvatum in a proximal tibial lengthening if not accounted for. The distal tibia may yield slower regenerate anteriorly because of a lack of soft tissue coverage. The nerves and vessels in general can adapt to gradual lengthening, but take 2 to 3 months to fully recover after distraction is completed.[16] Excessive gradual or acute distraction can yield nerve damage; given the distraction period is 4 to 8 times faster than adolescent growth spurts, surgeons must be cognitive of this.[11]

COMPLICATIONS

Distraction osteogenesis and bone transport are not without complications, including soft tissue scarring, muscle tethering, associated joint deformity, and pin tract inflammation or infection.[17] Patients will experience significant pain during distraction and consolidation. It may become necessary to stop lengthening for a period of time in distraction or slow distraction secondary to pain. Nerve injury or compartment syndrome can occur and should be identified early during lengthening. The stability of wires is essential in preventing pin irritation that may lead to infection. In addition, poor regenerate formation may occur for a multitude of reasons and can be dealt with by withdrawing or slowing distraction, dynamization techniques, or injecting BMA or PRP into the regenerate.[18] Lastly, an external fixator may take a psychological toll on patients, which should be discussed preoperatively.

CLINICS CARE POINTS

- Place corticotomy as close to metaphyseal bone as possible for vascularity.
- Latency period of 3 to 10 days is reported, but may be extended to 7 to 14 days if comorbidities are present.
- Distraction rate of 1 mm per day is most widely accepted; however, in the tibia with previous injury, slower daily rate may be more appropriate.
- External fixation removal is accepted with tricortical radiographic consolidation of the regenerate.
- Deformity and regenerate fracture are a few of many possible complications that can occur. Understanding of external fixation principles is critical.

DISCLOSURES

K. Millonig has nothing to disclose. B. Hutchinson has consulted for Orthofix.

REFERENCES

1. Ilizarov GA. The tension-stress effect on the genesis and growth of tissues: part II. The influence of the rate and frequency of distraction. Clin Orthop Relat Res 1989;239:263–85.
2. De Bastiani G, Aldegheri R, Renz-Brivio L, et al. Limb lengthening by callus distraction (callotasis). J Pediatr Orthop 1987;7:129–34.
3. Jeng CL, Campbell JT, Tang EY, et al. Tibiocalcaneal arthrodesis with bulk femoral head allograft for salvage of large defects in the ankle. Foot Ankle Int 2013;34(9):1256–66.
4. Sveshnikov AA, Barabash AP, Cheplenko TA, et al. Radionuclide studies of osteogenesis and circulation in substitution of large defects of the leg bones in experiment. Ortop Travmatol Protez 1984;11:33.
5. Ilizarov GA. Clinical application of the tension-stress effect for limb lengthening. Clin Orthop Relat Res 1990;250:8–26.
6. Delloye C, Delefortrie G, Coulter L, et al. Bone regenerate formation in cortical bone during distraction lengthening. an experimental study. Clin Orthop Relat Res 1990;250:34–42.
7. Cattaneo R, Villa A, Catagni MA, et al. Lengthening of the humerus using Ilizarov technique. Description of the method and report of 43 cases. Clin Orthop Relat Res 1990;250:117–24.
8. Green SA. Complications of external skeletal fixation. Clin Orthop Relat Res 1983; 180:109–16.

9. Paley D, Tetsworth K. Percutaneous osteotomies. Osteotome and Gigli saw techniques. Orthop Clin North Am 1991;22:613–24.

10. Lamm BM, Gourdine-Shaw MC, Thabet AM, et al. Distraction osteogenesis for complex foot deformities: gigli saw midfoot osteotomy with external fixation. J Foot Ankle Surg 2014;53(5):567–76.

11. Aronson J. Experimental and clinical experience with distraction osteogenesis. Cleft Palate Craniofac J 1994;31:473–81.

12. Bonnar C, Favard L, Sollogoub I, et al. Limb lengthening in children using the Ilizarov method. Clin Orthop Relat Res 1993;293:83–8.

13. Dahl MT, Gulli B, Berg T. Complications of limb lengthening. A learning curve. Clin Orthop Relat Res 1994;301:10–8.

14. Paley D. Current techniques of limb lengthening. J Pediatr Orthop 1988;8:73–92.

15. Fischgrund J, Paley D, Suter C. Variables affecting time to bone healing during limb lengthening. Clin Orthop Relat Res 1994;301:31–7.

16. Matano T, Tamai K, Kurokaea T. Adaptation of skeletal muscle in limb lengthening: a light diffraction study on the sarcomere length in situ. J Orthop Res 1994;12: 193–6.

17. Paley D. Problems, obstacles, and complications of limb lengthening by the Ilizarov technique. Clin Orthop 1990;250:81–104.

18. Lee DH, Ryu KJ, Kim JW, et al. Bone marrow aspirate concentrate and platelet-rich plasma enhanced bone healing in distraction osteogenesis of the tibia. Clin Orthop Relat Res 2014;472(12):3789–97.

The Free Fibula Flap for Lower Extremity Reconstruction

Christopher Bibbo, DO, DPM

KEYWORDS

- Fibula • Free flap • Bone defect • Tibia • Calcaneus • Foot • Adult • Pediatric

KEY POINTS

- The fibula as a free flap provides a large segment of vascularized bone.
- The fibula free flap blood supply in large part is derived from the muscular cuff and periosteum, which is nourished by the muscular branches of the peroneal artery.
- Bone defects from osteomyelitis, trauma, tumor, and congenital and acquired deformities are indications for the free fibula flap.
- Critical size defects and avascular bone beds of the femur, tibia, calcaneus, and foot may be successfully treated with the fibula free flap.
- External fixation after free fibula reconstruction provides patient mobilization and the ability to correct residual deformity.

INTRODUCTION

The fibula is an important resource for reconstructive purpose when used as a source of vascularized bone in musculoskeletal surgery with the best indications being the fibular transposition ("fibula-pro-tibia," "Huntington procedure"), reverse-pedicle myosseous flaps, but most importantly, fibula free flaps. The fibula is considered a relatively "expendable" bone, as it transmits only approximately 17% of body weight.[1] Traditionally, the proximal and distal syndesmotic articulations biomechanical functions were not fully appreciated (**Fig. 1**). However, musculoskeletal surgeons recognize that the distal tibial-fibular syndesmosis possesses complex biomechanical properties and is a critical structure for ankle stability. The ankle syndesmotic complex encompasses areas of the lateral and interosseous regions of the ankle, and extends well above the ankle joint line. For the ankle to function in a relatively normal fashion, the ankle syndesmosis must be preserved to a level as high as 7 cm above the ankle

Foot & Ankle Surgery, Plastic Reconstructive & Microsurgery, Orthopaedic Trauma and MSK Infection Services, Rubin Institute for Advanced Orthopedics, Sinai Hospital of Baltimore, 2401 West Belvedere Avenue, Baltimore, MD 21215, USA
E-mail address: drchrisbibbo@gmail.com

Clin Podiatr Med Surg 38 (2021) 117–130
https://doi.org/10.1016/j.cpm.2020.09.007
0891-8422/21/© 2020 Elsevier Inc. All rights reserved.

podiatric.theclinics.com

Donor Limb

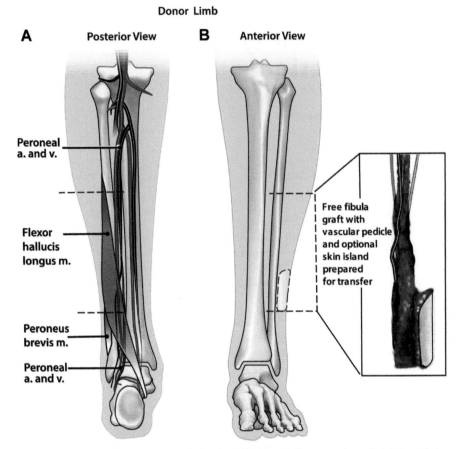

A   **Posterior View**   **B**   **Anterior View**

Peroneal
a. and v.

Flexor
hallucis
longus m.

Peroneus
brevis m.

Peroneal
a. and v.

Free fibula
graft with
vascular pedicle
and optional
skin island
prepared
for transfer

Fig. 1. Overview of the anatomy of the free fibula and flap template. (With Permission. Copyright 2020, Rubin Institute for Advanced Orthopedics, Sinai Hospital of Baltimore.)

joint line. The proximal tibiofibular syndesmosis is not as critical for limb function, but, the proximal 50% of fibular head is the attachment of the biceps femoris tendon and is part of the lateral stabilization mechanism of the knee. Thus, it is more accurate to state that most of the fibula is expendable, outside of the proximal and distal syndesmoses.

The anatomy and physiology of the fibula, as it relates to the use as a free flap, is unlike that of muscle or soft tissue; this holds for other bone free flaps such as the iliac crest, rib, and the medial femoral condyle. The nutrient vessel entering the bone is not necessarily the main source of blood supply when used as a free flap, as the nutrient vessel is excluded from the harvested flap. This is especially true with the free fibula flap, where the blood supply to the bone (outer cortex through to the medullary canal) is supplied via small vessels that traverse the periosteum, which in turn develop into fine vessels that perforate the cortex and traverse the cortex to the intramedullary space. These "periosteal cortical perforators" are direct branches from the intramuscular vessels of the flexor hallucis longus (FHL) muscle that branch off the peroneal artery (see **Fig. 1**; **Figs. 2–4**). The venous outflow of the fibula is via the medullary canal and what soft tissue present (muscle, skin) drains via the peroneal vein (see **Figs. 1**

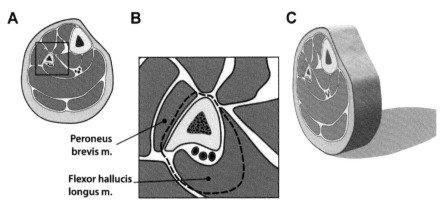

Peroneus
brevis m.

Flexor hallucis
longus m.

Fig. 2. Cross-sectional illustration of the leg and relationships of the pedicle and surrounding muscle. (With Permission. Copyright 2020, Rubin Institute for Advanced Orthopedics, Sinai Hospital of Baltimore.)

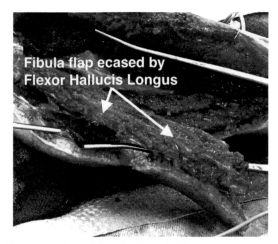

Fig. 3. Intraoperative photo highlighting the flexor hallucis longus surrounding the free fibula graft. Note the cuff of muscle left in situ and the skin island. (With Permission. Copyright 2020, Main Street Enterprises, LLC, DBA Global Medicus.)

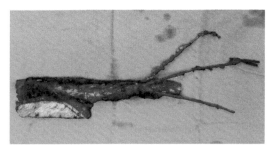

Fig. 4. Harvested free fibula osteocutaneous flap with artery (center, with "bulldog" clamp) and venae comitantes. (With Permission. Copyright 2020, Main Street Enterprises, LLC, DBA Global Medicus.)

and **4**). The peroneal artery provides muscular vessels to the FHL, which is the most important muscle that ensconces the fibula. Thus, to harvest a free fibula, the surgeon must take peroneal artery, the FHL in which it courses, and the fibula with FHL muscle firmly attached to the bone, all as one unit (see **Figs. 1–4**). The fibula provides a long length of bone (see **Fig. 4; Fig. 5**) and although of small diameter, has a triangular cross-section capable of withstanding high compressive and bending forces (see **Fig. 2**). Although thin, the fibula can over time provide greater girth via late hypertrophy (Wolff law).

CLINICAL INDICATIONS OF THE FIBULA FREE FLAP

Clinically, the free fibula may be used in the reconstruction of musculoskeletal defects associated with osteomyelitis (of various causes), trauma, tumors, congenital or acquired defects, as well as arthrodesis procedures (**Tables 1** and **2**). In the lower extremity, the free fibula is indicated when a critical size intercalary bone defect is present, that is otherwise unable to be reconstructed by conventional means. Critical size is defined in respect to the area of reconstruction. For example, a 5 cm is the end range of a critical size defect for the tibia,[2] whereas the author indicates a fibula free flap as a possible method for reconstruction for the foot columns (**Fig. 6**) and calcaneus (**Fig. 7**) when 3- to 4-cm defect exists in a poorly vascularized bed. Additional indications are to provide a source of blood supply to surrounding bone, such as in ankle fusions requiring structural vascularized bone as in widespread avascular necrosis. Another indication for the free fibula is when a defect requires a sufficient length

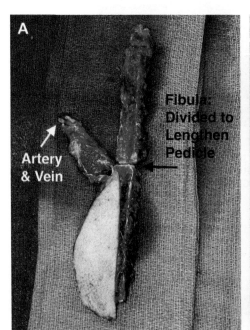
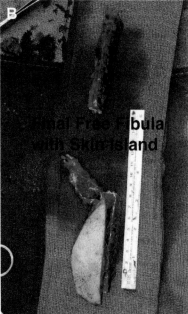

Fig. 5. (*A*) Intraoperative view of osteocutaneous free fibula flap. The near total length of fibula is harvested, then divided to maximize pedicle length. Note the generous cuff of the flexor hallucis muscle. (*B*) Final fibula free flap with skin island after division of excess bone. The excess bone may be used as well either intact or morselized. (With Permission. Copyright 2020, Main Street Enterprises, LLC, DBA Global Medicus.)

Table 1
Common uses of the fibula free flap for lower extremity reconstructions

	Knee	Tibia	Ankle	Hindfoot	Midfoot	Forefoot
PRIMARY INDICATIONS:	Fusions	Intercalary defects	Fusions	Fusions; talus & calcaneus defects	Fusions; bone defect	Intercalary defects
FREE FIBULA COMPOSITES:	Bone	Bone, often with skin	Bone, +/− skin.	Bone, rarely with skin	Bone, rarely with skin	Bone, rarely with skin

Table 2
Uses of proximal fibula physis free flap

Location	Purpose	Clinical Setting
Shoulder: proximal humerus	Longitudinal growth & maintain joint	Tumor
Wrist: distal radius	Longitudinal growth & maintain joint	Tumor
Hip: femoral head & neck	Longitudinal growth & maintain joint	Tumor
Ankle: distal fibula & lateral malleolus	Longitudinal growth, lateral buttress	Trauma

vascularized bone that also requires soft tissue ("skin") coverage of a wound—an osteocutaneous fibula free flap (see **Figs. 1, 4**, and **5**).

Pediatric indications for a free fibula flap are mostly for tibial and femoral reconstructions after trauma,[3] congenital pseudarthrosis of long bones,[4,5] and oncologic tumor resection.[6,7] The proximal fibula physis may also be used as a free flap. The indications for a proximal fibula physis free flap include reconstructions of the hip, shoulder, and wrist joints after tumor resection.[7] The pediatric proximal fibular physis free flap has also been successfully used as a free flap to create a stable vascularized, growing physis for pediatric tumor surgery and trauma (see **Table 2**). More recently, the pediatric physis free flap has been described to provide a vascularized physeal complex after severe pediatric ankle trauma, used to create a vascularized, growing lateral malleolus and ligaments.[8] The anatomic regions where a free fibula has application in the

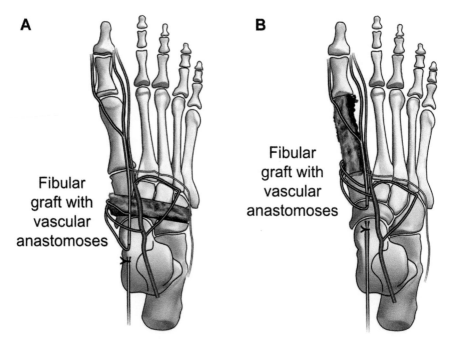

Fig. 6. The free fibula used to reconstruct the midfoot (*A*) and medial column (*B*). Vascular microanastomosis to a local source artery with the best access and vessel size match. (With Permission. Copyright 2020, Rubin Institute for Advanced Orthopedics, Sinai Hospital of Baltimore.)

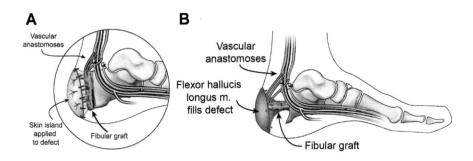

Fig. 7. (*A*) Application of the free fibula to reconstruct a vertical defect of the calcaneus and also providing posterior skin coverage of the heel. Note the microanastomotic pattern to the posterior tibial vessels. (*B*) The application of a free fibula with a large muscle cuff (osteomyocutaneous fibula free flap) to fill a posterior heel defect; this would then be covered with a skin graft. Note the microanastomotic pattern to the posterior tibial vessels. (With Permission. Copyright 2020, Rubin Institute for Advanced Orthopedics, Sinai Hospital of Baltimore.)

lower extremity from the knee to the foot are listed in **Table 1**. Uses of the pediatric proximal fibula physis free flap are listed in **Table 2**.

PREOPERATIVE EVALUATION

A critical first step in the reconstructive effort is an analysis of the surgical goal, such as limb preservation[9], functional joint preservation,[8] or the maintenance of a previous level of amputation,[10,11] which will determine the need for a free bone flap alone or a composite of bone with skin. Subsequently, the size of the osseous defect for the surgical goal must be expertly assessed using full length limb films (tibia), plain radiographs, and computed tomography (CT). The biomechanical requirements of the lower extremity region must also be evaluated to ascertain flap size requirements.

Competency of the vascular axis may be performed by Doppler examination. In the setting of pervious trauma, tumor resection, or multiple same-site surgeries, a CT angiography or angiogram is indicated. Adequacy of at least one other major vessel with sufficient collateralization must be present. Knowledge of the patient having a dominant peroneal artery with coexisting hypoplastic posterior tibial and anterior tibial arteries and the degree thereof are vital to preoperative planning. This anatomic variant exists in 5% of the population, with a 20% incidence of being bilateral.[12] The diagnosis of a peroneus arteries magna (0.5%)[12] is best made with arteriography and when present, prohibits free fibula harvest.

When managing infections, the infection site must be under control with adequate debridement's and culture-directed antibiotics. The formal algorithm for the evaluation and managing of osteomyelitis is beyond the scope of this article. An evaluation is made as to the need for adjunctive surgical procedures, such as external fixation[9] (**Fig. 8**), or in the case of a free fibula used in conjunction with an amputation, an immediate external fixation-based postoperative prosthesis (XProsthesis, PostOp Innovations, Fallston, MD)[12–15] (**Fig. 9**). Rehabilitation and social disposition issues are often overlooked in the preoperative planning process but are very important, as these may influence the overall surgical tactic. Including external fixation into the treatment plan may allow for improved rehabilitation and earlier hospital discharge.

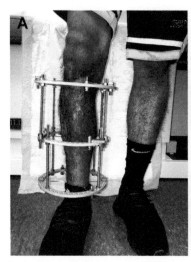 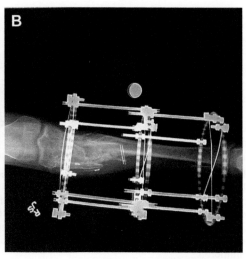

Fig. 8. (*A*) Patient who underwent a free fibula for a critical size traumatic tibial defect. Circular external fixation allows for early mobilization with progressive weight-bearing. The external fixator has been reduced over the course of time, gradually removed in the office. (*B*) Radiograph of the same patient in Fig. 8A, with a complete circular externa fixator, later scaled back. Because of the proximity of the defect, as well as severe fibrosis, a transposition flap (Huntington procedure) could not be performed. Note the K-wires to hold the ipsilateral free fibula bone flap in place. Residual deformity correction may be completed during healing at a later date with a hexapod external fixation system (Hexapod, OrthoFix, Plano, Texas). (With Permission. Copyright 2020, Main Street Enterprises, LLC, DBA Global Medicus.)

SURGICAL TECHNIQUE

The patient is positioned supine, with a hip "bump" to rotate the lateral leg into view. The knee may be flexed. A tourniquet may speed dissection but may prolong time to achieve hemostasis after harvest; thus, a "wet dissection" is frequently used. The proximal extent of ankle syndesmosis is marked clinically or radiographically. The neck of the fibula and course of the common peroneal nerve are outlined. If a skin island is desired, the distal septal perforating vessels are identified with a Doppler and marked with sutures; the skin island is designed based on defect size and location.

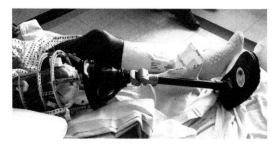

Fig. 9. The XProsthesis (PostOp Innovations, Fallston MD) used for immediate weight-bearing in major lower extremity amputations. This device is also applicable to protect free fibula grafts used to heal intercalary gone defects and maintain level of amputation. (With Permission. Copyright 2020, Main Street Enterprises, LLC, DBA Global Medicus.)

Skin islands are most reliable in the distal leg above the ankle syndesmosis; most skin island donor sites will need skin grafting.

The first operative step is identification and standard microvascular preparation of the recipient vessels. In instances of chronic wounds and bone defects, this step may be the most tedious and most time consuming. Recipient vessel preparation must maximize available artery and veins for anastomosis and lay in a "friendly" soft tissue bed.

A linear incision is made along the length of the proximal and distal limb, only exposing the fibular neck and lateral malleolus if needed (**Fig. 10**). The lateral aspect of the fibula is identified, and the peroneus brevis muscle completely elevated of the fibula—a cuff of peroneal muscle and periosteum is left on the lateral surface of the fibula—this is very important. The superficial peroneal nerve is left undisturbed. Dissection continues into the anterior compartment, sweeping the anterior musculature off the interosseous membrane (IOM). The IOM is split longitudinally; the FHL muscle is now exposed.

Distally, the peroneal artery and vein are identified behind the fibula, ligated, and divided at the desired level of fibular division distally (just above the most proximal extent of the syndesmotic complex). The fibula is then osteotomized distally, protecting the vessels with a ribbon retractor; a small suture should be placed to secure the vessels and surrounding soft tissue to the periosteal sleeve. The author recommends syndesmotic screw fixation, especially in young patients, at this moment or just before closure. Dissection proceeds from distal to proximal; maintaining a generous cuff of FHL muscle around the entire fibula is mandatory (see **Figs. 1, 4,** and **5**), as FHL muscle houses the peroneal vessels (see **Fig. 2**) and is the sentinel portion of the technique for elevating a free fibula graft.

Dissection proceeds to the tibioperoneal trunk—the proximity of this is often marked by a large "rats nest" of veins. This may confuse the course of the peroneal artery projection off its source vessels. When the peroneal origin is approached, the surgeon must determine if there exists a peronea arteria magna (0.5% of the population),[12] which would be the sole blood supply to the limb—the procedure would need to be abandoned. If there exists a very dominant peroneal artery and hypoplastic posterior and anterior tibial arteries (5% of the population; 20% of these are bilateral),[12] the contralateral limb may be used or the surgeon be prepared, if needed, to perform a double bypass with long reverse saphenous vein graft harvested from both limbs (not recommended except for the most experienced surgeon). This scenario is a reason for preoperative identification of this anatomic variant.

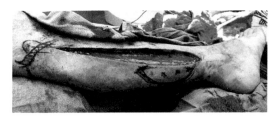

Fig. 10. Incision placement for the free fibula in relation to the common peroneal nerve and ankle syndesmosis. Note the skin island design accommodating the skin perforators that emanate from behind the fibula; the posterior incision for the skin island is executed last, being certain to include the vessels within the skin island. (With Permission. Copyright 2020, Main Street Enterprises, LLC, DBA Global Medicus.)

Next, the fibula is divided below the common peroneal nerve. By rotating the fibula shaft laterally, visualization of the vessels is maximized. Division of the peroneal vessels is performed as high as possible. Proximally, the source peroneal vessels are doubly ligated by hand or clips, and the open ends of the peroneal vessels on the flap are separated (see **Fig. 4**), then thoroughly flushed with heparinized saline solution (5000 units per 100 cc normal saline) until the vessels fluid runs clear. All side veins coming off the peroneal veins must be sealed with microclips.

The fibula is then trimmed with extreme care at its proximal end to create a longer vascular pedicle as needed (see **Fig. 5**). The fibula may be divided with a hinge at half its length and folded on itself to create a shorter but thicker bone graft (double barrel fibula, **Fig. 11**). Custom 3-dimensional printed cutting blocks are available for various cuts in the fibula but are mostly used for mandibular reconstruction—they are expensive and in general fibula cuts are simple; these devices are rarely used in lower extremity reconstruction. An implantable microvascular Doppler monitor may be placed if desired. After microvascular anastomosis of the artery and vein, the fibula is carefully inset and may be secured to the recipient bone by plate osteosynthesis or Kirschner-wire fixation. Regardless of the fixation method, implants must be placed on a surface of the fibula that is away from the pedicle, and, screw tips must not be

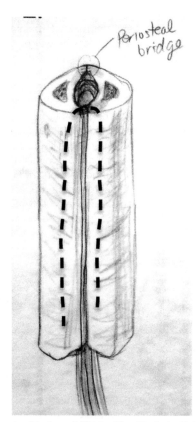

Fig. 11. Artist sketch of a double-barrel fibula. The fibula is divided and doubled on itself (blue *line*) hinged on a periosteal hinge. (With Permission. Copyright 2020, Rubin Institute for Advanced Orthopedics, Sinai Hospital of Baltimore.)

proud. In-setting may be accomplished with a simple on-lay, interposition, or inset via a trough. A "peg-in-hole" technique allows for a custom fit, and when performed an extra 1 to 2 cm of fibula must be designed into the final flap to create the bone "pegs." Microanastomosis is performed with 8-0 nylon, end-side arterial and end-end venous (**Fig. 12**). The question of whether vein anastomosis is necessary is considered controversial by some, unless a skin island is included in which case a venous anastomosis is mandatory (see **Figs. 1–5, 7, 8**, and **11**).

Accompanying external fixation may be either a pin-to-bar construct, circular rings with skinny wires or half-pins (see **Fig. 8**), or a transition protocol form the former to the latter. An external fixation protocol for ambulation or correction of a residual limb deformity is extremely valuable when the free fibula is used in tibial reconstructions.[9] When the free fibula is used for fusions or to reconstruct bone loss of the foot columns or calcaneus (see **Figs. 6** and **7**), the author prefers a fine wire circular external fixator with rapid adjust struts (TruLok, OrthoFix, Plano Texas) as described in his "flap and frame" technique.[13,14]

Postoperatively, the reconstructed part is elevated without circumferential or any snug dressings. Vessel patency is monitored by Doppler signal of skin island perforator, implantable Doppler devices, or over the anastomosis site marked externally. The author's postoperative protocol mirrors that of soft tissue flaps (**Box 1**). Strict physical therapy orders (Figure Legend—) with full weight-bearing on a contralateral

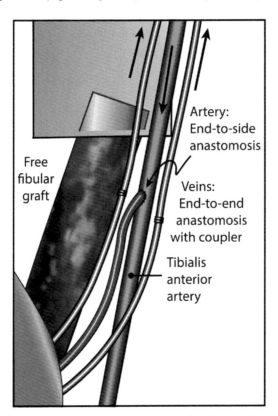

Fig. 12. Close-up illustrative view of the end-side arterial and end-end venous microanastomoses for a free fibula graft. Venous couplers are depicted. (With Permission. Copyright 2020, Rubin Institute for Advanced Orthopedics, Sinai Hospital of Baltimore.)

Box 1
Generalized free flap postoperative protocols: postoperative orders, dangling, discharge instructions

POD #0

NPO, start of Q 1 hour flap check for 48 hours postop (typically in ICU).

Urine output must be greater than ½ cc per kg per hour for 48 hours postop, IVF boluses if decreases less than threshold.

Laboratories: BMP, CBC in recovery based on intraoperative course.

Radiographs in recovery room.

POD #1

Clear liquid diet; OOB to chair strict elevation & strict NWB; resume home medications except for diuretics (do NOT give furosemide unless patient has severe fluid overload). Continue to monitor flap and urine output.

Laboratories: BMP, CBC.

POD #2

Advance to regular diet, double portions, protein supplements with each meal.

D/C Foley in PM if able, decrease IVF, start PO narcotics.

Q 2-hour flap check starts AFTER 48 hours postop.

Laboratories: BMP, CBC.

POD #3

Heplock IVF, full diet with protein supplements. Rehabilitation evaluation and discharge planning for discharge needs and therapy.

Laboratories: BMP, CBC.

POD #4/5

D/C to home (soft tissue flaps). Q 4-hour flap checks if remains in hospital.

Radiographs.

Anticoagulation:

Enoxaparin, 30 mg, SQ BID or Heparin 5000 units SQ Q 8 hours; ASA, 325 mg, PO QD x4 weeks at discharge.

Resume anti-factor Xa drugs on case to case basis; preferably POD #5 to 7.

Lower Extremity Dangle Protocols:
A. Minimal Limb Edema:
  - Dangle on POD#7 & #8 for 15 minutes Q 6 hours; POD #9 & #10 for 30 minutes Q 6 hours; POD#11 & 12 for 45 minutes Q 6 hours; POD#13 for 60 minutes Q 6 hours
B. Acute or Chronic Limb Edema:
  - Start dangle POD #14 to 16 dangle for 15 minutes Q 6 hours; POD # 17 to 18 for 30 minutes Q 6 hours; POD # 19 to 21 for 45 minutes Q 6 hours; POD# 22 for 60 minutes Q 6 hours

---

Discharge Instructions of Free Flap Patients:

Medications: antibiotics—first-generation cephalosporin x1week, or, per infectious disease recommendation for infected cases; aspirin, 325 mg, PO QD x4 weeks; low-dose narcotics PRN; gabapentin, 300 mg, PO TID x4 weeks.

Discharge activity: individualized prescription based on fibula flap location, intercalary defect versus fusion.

Discuss postoperative orders with collaborating services and nursing. Orders are modified based on individual case needs. Bone-only flaps may have accelerated schedules.

---

donor limb are ordered; occupational therapy for upper extremity strengthening. Discharge planning is commenced early.

A weight-bearing protocol is individualized based on the reconstructive sight. The author obtains intraoperative radiographs, repeated at 7 days, on first clinic visit, then every 4 to 8 weeks. A CT is obtained when full weight-bearing is being planned to ensure appropriate level of bone consolidation. The bone flap requires a form of protective prosthetic, such as an off-loading ankle foot orthosis, whereas the graft continues to mature. Discontinuation of any prosthetic appliance merits a repeat CT to document satisfactory bone healing.

Discharge care plays an important role in the success of any flap reconstruction. Patient nutrition plans mirror that of when in the hospital. Smoking, vaping, and alcohol are prohibited. Showering (not soaking) is permitted as soon as suture lines are "sealed or "healed," usually at 14 to 21 days using a gentle soap. Incisions may have antibiotic ointment applied and covered with a dry dressing as needed. Edema wraps are permitted at 3 to 4 weeks. Weeping edema should be dressed to soak-up fluids and changed as needed to keep the leg dry. Skin conditioning is permitted with a fragrance-free, water-based cream.

SUMMARY

The fibula free flap is the most common source of vascularized bone for the reconstruction of complex, critical size bone defects in the lower extremity. These locations include the femur, tibia, calcaneus, and foot columns and midfoot. The free fibula may also be used in arthrodesis procedures. The free fibula may carry a skin island for flap monitoring, and when well designed, the skin island may provide coverage of defects of the soft tissue envelope.

DISCLOSURE

The author has nothing to disclose.

REFERENCES

1. Lambert KL. The weight-bearing function of the fibula. A strain gauge study. J Bone Joint Surg Am 1971;53(3):507–13.
2. Malizos KN, Zalavras CG, Soucacos PN, et al. Free vascularized fibular grafts for reconstruction of skeletal defects. J Am Acad Orthop Surg 2004;12(5):360–9.
3. Momeni A, Lanni M, Levin LS, et al. Microsurgical reconstruction of traumatic lower extremity defects in the pediatric population. Plast Reconstr Surg 2017; 139(4):998–1004.

4. Iamaguchi RB, Fucs PM, Carlos da Costa A, et al. Congenital pseudoarthrosis of the tibia – results of treatment by free fibular transfer and associated procedures – preliminary study. J Pediatr Orthop B 2011;20(5):323–9.

5. Gilbert A, Brockman R. Congenital pseudarthrosis of the tibia. Long-term follow-up of 29 cases treated by microvascular bone transfer. Clin Orthop Relat Res 1995;(314):37–44.

6. Ghoneimy AME, Sherbiny ME, Kamal N. Use of vascularized fibular free flap in the reconstruction of the femur in pediatric and adolescent bone sarcomas: complications and functional outcome. J Reconstr Microsurg 2019;35(2):156–62.

7. Innocenti M, Ceruso M, Manfrini M, et al. Free vascularized growth-plate transfer after bone tumor resection in children. J Reconstr Microsurg 1998;14(2):137–43.

8. Bibbo C, Mayer BE, Michetti LA. Foot and ankle surgery for chronic non-healing wounds. Surg Clin North Am 2020;100(4):707–25. https://doi.org/10.1016/j.suc.2020.05.003.

9. Bibbo C, Bauder A, Nelson J, et al. Reconstruction of traumatic tibia defects with free fibula flap and external fixation. Ann Plast Surg 2020. https://doi.org/10.1097/SAP.0000000000002240.

10. Bibbo C, Ehrlich DA, Kovach SJ. Pediatric lateral ankle physeal reconstruction by free microvascular transfer of the proximal fibular physis. J Foot Ankle Surg 2015;54(5):994–1000.

11. Bibbo C, Ehrlich D, Levin LS, et al. Maintaining levels of lower extremity amputations. J Surg Orthop Adv 2016;25(3):137–48.

12. Bibbo C, Kovack SJ, Mehta S, et al. General principles of limb salvage versus amputation in adults. In: Krajbich JI, Pinzur MS, Potter BK, et al, editors. Atlas of amputations and limb deficiencies. 4th edition. Chicago: America Academy of Orthopaedic Surgeons; 2016. p. 41–59. Chapter 4.

13. Abou-Foul AK, Borumandi F. Anatomical variants of lower limb vasculature and implications for free fibula flap: Systematic review and critical analysis. Microsurgery 2016;36(2):165–72.

14. Bibbo C. A novel limb salvage technique of external fixation protection of lower extremity plastic reconstructions with immediate post-operative ambulation ("Bibbo Flap & Frame Technique"). Clin Podiatr Med Surg 2021;38(1):55–71.

15. Bibbo C. The use of an external fixator coupled immediate post-operative prosthesis (X-Prosthesis) after major lower extremity amputation. Clinics Podiatric Medicine & Surgery, in press.

Printed and bound by CPI Group (UK) Ltd, Croydon, CR0 4YY

03/10/2024

01040402-0014